HOT TOPICS IN BURN INJURIES

Edited by **Selda Pelin Kartal**
and **Dilek Bayramgürler**

Hot Topics in Burn Injuries
http://dx.doi.org/10.5772/intechopen.69253
Edited by Selda Pelin Kartal and Dilek Bayramgürler

Contributors

Allison Cowin, Xanthe Strudwick, Mehmet Unal, Pertevniyal Bodamyalızade, Serap Maden, Emel Çalıkoğlu, Yeşim Akpınar Kara, Selda Pelin Kartal, Cemile Tuba Altunel, Dilek Bayramgurler

First published in London, United Kingdom, 2018 by IntechOpen
IntechOpen is the global imprint of INTECHOPEN LIMITED, registered in England and Wales, registration number: 11086078, The Shard, 25th floor, 32 London Bridge Street
London, SE19SG – United Kingdom
Printed in Croatia

British Library Cataloguing-in-Publication Data
A catalogue record for this book is available from the British Library

Additional hard copies can be obtained from orders@intechopen.com

Hot Topics in Burn Injuries, Edited by Selda Pelin Kartal and Dilek Bayramgürler
p. cm.
Print ISBN 978-1-78923-130-4
Online ISBN 978-1-78923-131-1

For EU product safety concerns:
IN TECH d.o.o., Prolaz Marije Krucifikse Kozulić 3, 51000 Rijeka, Croatia,
info@intechopen.com or visit our website at intechopen.com.

Meet the editors

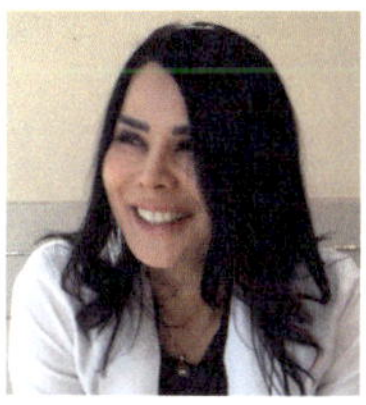

Assoc. Prof. Dr. Selda Pelin Kartal graduated from the Hacettepe University Faculty of Medicine. Currently, she is an associate professor at the Department of Dermatology of the University of Health Sciences, Dişkapi Yildirim Beyazit Training and Research Hospital in Ankara, Turkey. She has coauthored over 100 published articles and supervised several master's and postdoctoral students. Her interests focus on acne, psoriasis, urticaria, autoimmune bullous diseases, Behçet's disease, hair disorders, burn injury and cosmetic dermatology.

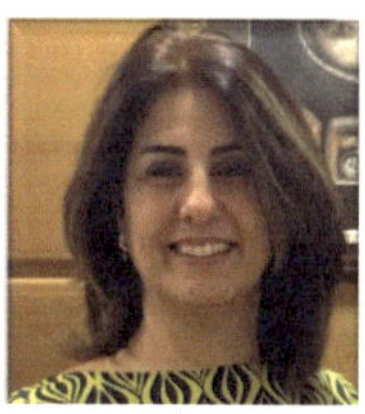

Prof. Dr. Dilek Bayramgürler graduated from the Marmara University School of Medicine. Currently, she is a professor at the Department of Dermatology of the Kocaeli University Faculty of Medicine in Kocaeli, Turkey. She has coauthored nearly 100 published articles. Cutaneous lymphomas, phototherapy, acne and psoriasis are her main interests in the field of dermatology.

Contents

Preface

The aim of this book is to give readers a broad review of burn injuries, which may affect people from birth to death and can lead to high morbidity and mortality.

The book consists of four sections and seven chapters. The first section consists of the introductory review chapter, which overviews the burn injuries. The second section includes chapter "Burn Etiology and Pathogenesis," which focuses on burn injuries and clinical findings. The third section consists of chapter "Controlling Inflammation in Burn Injury" and is devoted to the role of inflammatory response, which is fundamental to the healing process, while a prolonged inflammation may lead to scarring and fibrosis. The fourth section consists of four chapters as follows: "Therapeutic Effects of Conservative Treatments on Burn Scars," "Herbal Therapy for Burns and Burn Scars," "Platelet-Rich Plasma in Burn Treatment," and "Surgical Treatment of Burn Scars."

We are grateful to all the contributors and leading experts for the submission of their wonderful work that provides an in-depth view of all aspects of the content, backed with the most current literature in the field. We offer our special thanks and appreciation to Ms. Kristina Kardum, Publishing Process Manager, for her encouragement and help in bringing out the book in the present form and to our families for their understanding for missed family time.

We express our heartfelt gratitude to great Atatürk, who said "Our true mentor in life is science" and inspired the importance of working on positive science.

Assoc. Prof. Dr. Selda Pelin Kartal
Ministry of Health Ankara
Dişkapı Yildirim Beyazit Training and Research Hospital Dermatology Clinic
Ankara, Turkey

Prof. Dr. Dilek Bayramgürler
Kocaeli University
Department of Dermatology
Kocaeli, Turkey

Section 1

General Description of Burn Injuries

Chapter 1

Introductory Chapter: An Introduction to Burn Injuries

Selda Pelin Kartal, Cemile Tuğba Altunel and
Dilek Bayramgurler

Additional information is available at the end of the chapter

http://dx.doi.org/10.5772/intechopen.71973

1. Introduction

Burn injury of the skin is characterized by the damage to skin tissue from hot (scald, flash, flame, contact), cold, electrical, chemical, radiation, sunlight, or other sources. Burns constitute one of the most common causes of morbidity and mortality worldwide. They can result in significant disfigurement, physical impairment, work loss, psychological problems, and considerable economic burden. Prevention of burn is considered the best strategy to reduce the overall burden of burns. The impact and the management of burn injury depend on the severity of burn. Although minor burns can be treated at outpatient clinics, the management of patients with severe burns requires multidisciplinary approach in specialized burn care centers. Burn trauma differs from the other causes of injuries in many aspects. Increased knowledge about the pathophysiology of burn provided better treatment plans and led to the improvement of overall outcome for these patients. Formation of scar is an undesired consequence of burn with many long-term complications. The local treatment of burn wound should address the major concerns of wound care including anti-inflammatory treatment, wound coverage, and prevention of infection and scar formation. Although superficial burns may be managed with topical treatment, deep burns require excision and grafting. As traditional treatments have many limitations, alternative options with better outcomes have been searched in the restoration of damaged tissues. Tissue-engineered products, stem cells, and gene therapy constitute new concepts that offer promise in the treatment of burn wounds. Although the results with these innovations are encouraging, they require sophisticated techniques, and evidence for their long-term efficacy in burn wounds is lacking. Future search will introduce novel therapeutic options and assist in the establishment of standard burn wound care in clinical settings [1–3].

2. Epidemiology of burn injuries and risk factors for burns

Burns constitute a major health problem worldwide. Considerable amount of patients suffer or die from burn injuries globally. The burns mostly occur in low- and middle-income regions of the world [1, 4, 5]. Burn injuries occur more commonly in men at young adult age [5–8]; however, in elderly, female predominance is seen [5, 6, 8]. Alcohol usage, smoking, presence of open fire source or ground level stoves, wearing high-risk cloths (long, loose-fitting, synthetic), improper temperature setting of water heaters, use of unsafe electrical equipment, use of kerosene lamps, low socioeconomic status, overpopulation, illiteracy, unemployment, belonging to a large and single-parent family, and housing without adequate health and safety requirements are all reported to be risk factors for burn injury [4, 7, 9, 10].

3. Severity of burn injuries

Fortunately, most of the burn injuries fall into mild cases that can be treated in community or in outpatient clinics. However, depending on the severity of the condition, hospitalization or treatment in intensive care unit may be needed [5, 6, 8]. Severity of a burn injury depends on the extent of burned area (expressed as the percentage of total body surface area (TBSA)), depth of tissue damage, presence or absence of inhalation injury, mechanism of injury, age of the patient, and accompanying comorbidities [8]. Median TBSA of all burn cases was reported as 15%, and severe burn injuries constitute less than 10% of total burns [5, 6, 8]. Mostly children, women, and elderly people are affected by severe burns. Low socioeconomic status and being from ethnic minorities are considered as risk factors for experiencing severe burns [5]. Inhalation injury is seen in less than 4% of cases and more likely to be observed in extensive burns [8].

4. Etiology of burn injuries

Burn injuries can result from diverse etiologies including flames, scalds, contact, electricity, chemicals, or even sunlight. The mechanism may differ according to the sex, age, residence, ethnicity, and admittance status (admitted or non-admitted) of the patient. In general, scald, flame, and contact are the major mechanisms for burns [5–7, 10]. Electrical and chemical burns occur less frequently. Other than the abovementioned mechanisms, many other causes including sunburn and flash lasers can also result in burn injury [5].

5. Mortality from burn injuries

Mortality rate from burn injuries differs among different studies and is reported between 1.4 and 18% [5, 6]. Older age, high extent of burned surface, concomitant illnesses, the presence of inhalation injury, African-American race, urban practice setting, and facial location of burn are all considered as risk factors for mortality [5–8, 10]. Flame burns are in general more fatal than contact burns. Mortality from burn injury is most commonly related to multiorgan failure and sepsis. Pneumonia and acute respiratory distress syndrome (ARDS) are also associated with mortality [5, 8, 11].

6. Ethical issues

In all, but especially pediatric and elderly burns, legal and ethical issues should be considered. As abuse and maltreatment may go unnoticed, identification of suspicious injuries by the physician is important. Delayed referral, suspicious and unreliable history, inconsistent explanations of parents or caregivers, tap water injury, and the presence of immersion lines are some of the clues that should raise the suspicion of abuse [3, 12, 13].

7. Precautions for burn patients

As most of the burns occur accidentally, prevention strategies remain the best approach in order to reduce the morbidity and mortality associated with burns. Increasing knowledge about the epidemiology of burn injuries will aid in defining preventable risk factors that should be targeted. While safety interventions for work-related burns decrease the risk, certain cultural practices and social habits may be related with increased burn accidents in certain geographic regions. Although education and increased awareness of public play important roles in prevention strategies, the introduction of legislation and better regulations are more effective in reducing the burn injury. Additionally, enforcement of legislation is critical to increase the success of prevention programs [5, 9, 10].

8. Pathophysiology of burn wounds

Systemic nature of the burn injury is unique that should be taken into consideration while approaching the patient. Understanding the pathophysiology of burn will provide useful information for early and effective management of burn patients, improve the quality of care for burn wounds, allow the identification of novel targets for the treatment of scar formation, and contribute to efforts to reduce the mortality. The local burn wound induces a generalized inflammatory response characterized by the activation of cytokines and release of various growth factors that can result in detrimental effects on many organs. The magnitude of this response depends on the severity of burn [1, 3, 5, 14, 15]. One of the distinct features of burn injury is that the cytokine-mediated signaling triggered by the tissue damage results in a generalized increase in capillary permeability and extravasation of plasma causing exaggerated edema response even at distant sites [3, 15]. Loss of intravascular fluid is accompanied by a decrease in cardiac output and increase in peripheral vascular resistance that may lead to hypoperfusion of organs and burn shock [1, 3, 15]. Hypercoagulability may occur due to systemic activation of platelet aggregation and fibrinolysis [1]. After the edema phase, a hypermetabolic state ensues which is characterized by an increase in oxygen consumption, marked protein and lipid catabolism, increase in energy requirements, high cardiac output, tachycardia, severe muscle weakness, cachexia, and decrease in immune functions [3, 15, 16].

Although the wound healing phases are similar to other types of wounds, the prolonged healing time is especially important in burn wounds [1–3]. The severity of burn, the mechanism of injury, and associated diseases of patients influence the wound healing [1]. Inflammatory phase includes the vasodilation and inflammatory cell migration through the cytokine signaling cascade. In proliferative phase, epithelization takes place by the migration of keratinocytes from the epithelium of the wound edges and dermal appendages. Remodeling (maturation) phase is characterized by the deposition of collagen by myofibroblasts, compaction of the connective tissue, and finally the contraction of the wound. Although the wound contraction and scar formation are normal and necessary for the closure of wound, excessive fibrosis and increased tensile stress during remodeling carry the risk of abnormal scar formation. Intense and prolonged inflammatory response with increased release of cytokines, growth factors, and other mediators from the inflammatory cells and platelets are associated with scar formation. The depth of burn, age of the patient, the treatment, and response of wound are important determinants for the development of scar tissue. Wounds that are not healed in 2–3 weeks are generally at risk of developing aberrant scar tissue [1–3].

Superficial burn wounds heal completely in 5–7 days during the proliferative phase. As the required dermal components are lost in deep burns, proliferation cannot be provided, and the epithelialization is delayed. The lack of supportive and vascular tissue is associated with abnormal contraction, and these wounds heal with hypertrophic scarring and contractures if left to heal spontaneously [1–3].

9. Management of the burn patient at first step

Early and appropriate treatment of burn injury is associated with better prognosis. Prehospital management and the treatment of burn patients in the emergency department fall out of the scope of this chapter and include the general rules for trauma patients. As the airway edema may start soon after burn and unexpectedly, early intubation may be indicated. Since massive edema may develop in extended burns, all jewelry and accessories should be taken off. Specific interventions may be indicated according to the mechanism of burn (electrical, chemical burns). Until the patient is referred to the medical center, wounds should just be covered with clean cloth. Cooling with compress may be done; however, unburned regions should be kept warm in order to avoid hypothermia [12, 15].

As the hypovolemic shock is associated with high morbidity and mortality, fluid resuscitation should be done early and adequately. Several criteria have been described for fluid resuscitation of burn patients [11, 17].

10. Evaluation of the severity of burn and referral of the patient

Assessing the severity of burn injury is important in deciding the need for hospitalization. To assess the severity of damage, special indexes have been described including "Burn Index (BI)" and "prognostic burn index (PBI)" [11].

To assess the extent of burned area, several methods can be used including rule of nines, rule of fives, and Lund-Browder Chart. Lund-Browder Chart is especially used for children which more accurately estimates the age-specific percentage of TBSA [11, 12, 15]. Additionally, for local assessments of small burns, the palm method (palm with fingers accounts for 1% of total body surface area) can be used practically in adults. First-degree burns are not considered in the calculation of TBSA [11, 12].

Although more precise methods including laser Doppler flowmetry and video microscopy have been defined, the depth of burn is mostly estimated clinically (the presence of pain or blister, appearance and color of the skin) in practice [11, 15]. Burns can be classified into three types according to the depth of injury:

(a) **First degree (superficial):** Only the epidermis is involved. The skin is red and painful. There is usually no blistering and skin will blanch when touched. It heals without scarring.

(b) **Second degree (partial thickness):** In superficial dermal burns (SDB), only the papillary dermis is involved. In this case the skin is painful. Blisters are seen. When the bullae are deroofed, the skin is wet and blanches when touched. It heals with minimal pigmentary changes without hypertrophic scarring. If the reticular dermis is involved, it is considered as deep dermal burn (DDB). In this case, there is less pain and no bullae or blistering. There is eschar and the skin is white or yellow. It does not blanch on pressure. It heals with scarring.

(c) **Third degree (full thickness):** There is little or no pain. It involves the epidermis and dermis and extends to the subcutaneous layer. The skin is leathery, dark, and inelastic. There is eschar. It does not blanch. It does not heal spontaneously, results in hypertrophic scar and contractures, and requires grafting [3, 11, 12].

Fourth-degree burns involve deeper structures including the subcutaneous tissue, muscle, tendons, ligaments, and bone. There is gangrene of tissue and carbonized appearance [12].

After the prehospital stabilization of the patient, depending on the severity of injury, treatment in a more equipped hospital may be required [11, 12]. The referral criteria may vary across different studies. To explain roughly, while major burns must be managed in hospitals with multidisciplinary burn teams, moderate burns can be managed in minor hospitals. No matter the extent, chemical burns, burns due to lighting strike, burns during pregnancy, and burns with suspicion of child abuse must be hospitalized. On the other hand, minor burns can be treated at outpatient clinics [3, 11, 12].

Pain management is important in burn patients since the discomfort from pain results in anxiety, increases the risk of prolonged hospitalization, leads to loss of patient confidence, and complicates the interventional procedures [12, 18]. Burn patients may suffer from different types of pain including background and procedural pain. In severe burns, moderate to potent opioids (fentanyl, morphine, ketamine, and others) are preferred, and non-steroidal anti-inflammatory drugs (NSAIDs) may be added to reduce the overall dose of opioids. NSAIDs may be sufficient to relieve pain in patients with mild to moderate burns. As they reduce the perception of pain, anxiolytics such as benzodiazepines may also be used. Although mild anesthetics are adequate for simple procedures, deeper anesthesia (with tramadol, ketamine, etc.) is required for the patients with severe burns during excision and grafting. Antidepressants and anticonvulsants are used as first-line therapies for neuropathic pain that may be seen in burn patients. Psychological therapies have also been reported with various successes for management of pain [12, 18].

11. Local treatment of burn wounds

Knowing the mechanisms involved in wound healing is very important for effective treatment of burn wounds. The treatment strategy for the burn wound varies according to the extent and depth of injury [1–3].

11.1. Burn wound care at first step and emergency department

Interventions that should be done at first step may differ according to the severity and mechanism of the burn. For minor burns, burned area should be put under running tap water for 20 min. Clothing that are soaked in hot liquid or contaminated with chemicals should be removed. For chemical burns, neutralizing agents should not be applied (neutralization reaction may cause further heat). Dry chemicals should be brushed away first and then irrigated with tap water. Before transfer to the designated facility, wounds should be wrapped with clean cloth but not covered with topical drugs. Topical silver sulfadiazine can be applied initially at the emergency department except for facial burns. Topical anesthetics are not recommended. Adherent dressings should not be used. Irrigation should be done with caution in order to avoid hypothermia due to cold water exposure [12]. As mentioned above, depending on the severity of burn, wound care in a multidisciplinary burn center may be required [11, 12, 15].

11.2. Topics to be covered in burn wound treatment

As previously mentioned, prolonged and exaggerated inflammatory response in deep burns results in intensified edema which further delays wound repair and is associated with scarring. Although the anti-inflammatory treatments such as prostaglandin inhibitors and glucocorticoids carry the risk of impaired wound healing, it seems reasonable to diminish excess inflammation and edema in burn injury [2, 19]. Indeed, treatment with topical or low dose systemic glucocorticoids in the early phase of burns has been suggested to prevent aberrant inflammation [11, 20]. For deep burns, early excision and grafting are crucial to remove the foci of inflammation and infection. Anti-inflammatory drugs including cytokine inhibitors, corticosteroids, interferons α and β, and methotrexate have also been used to prevent scar formation [1].

As the infection risk is increased in burn patients due to immunosuppression and the wounds can be rapidly contaminated by the organisms, prevention of infection should be the primary strategy in burn wound care [3, 11, 12]. Disinfectants can be used without inhibiting wound healing, and wounds should be cleaned with tap water, saline, and non-irritant soaps [11, 12]. Early covering of burn wound with topical antimicrobial agents may prevent the invasion or contamination of wound [3]. In deep burns, microorganisms may colonize the tissue below the eschar producing a source for infection. As the standard topical antimicrobials cannot penetrate the eschar tissue, early excision of the eschar is important in prevention of infection. Furthermore, early detection of infection is crucial especially in patients with deep and extensive burns [1–3]. Prophylactic antibiotics are not recommended for burn wounds unless there is high probability of infection. In case of wound contamination and in immunocompromised patients (pediatric, perioperative, and diabetic patients), prophylactic antibiotics can be considered [11, 12].

As the burn injury results in a profound hypermetabolic state, nutritional support is recommended in order to enhance wound healing [2, 3, 21]. Although the periodical clinical examination of the wound by the specialist stays the primary way of tracking wound healing, simple measurement tools, sophisticated techniques, and various serum parameters can be used to predict the likelihood of healing and for the follow-up of improvement in healing [2, 22, 23].

11.3. Burn wound coverage and grafting

11.3.1. For the first-degree burn wounds

For the first-degree wounds, topical antibiotics are not necessary. Moisturizing agents are sufficient, and topical anesthetics may be given depending on the patient's condition [12].

11.3.2. For superficial second-degree burn wounds

Although the burn wounds are sterile at the beginning of injury, the wound begins to be invaded by the organisms from the patient's flora or from the environment. Therefore, topical antimicrobials are recommended for superficial second-degree burn wounds. As silver sulfadiazine delays epithelialization, it can be used only for the first days to prevent infection. Wounds should be covered with non-adherent dressings including paraffin-impregnated gauze or ointments containing 0.2% nitrofurazone, zinc oxide, or dimethyl isopropylazulene. Several alternative topical agents have also been suggested to be effective [12]. Various types of dressing materials are available for the local care of burn wounds. Wound dressing selection should be tailored according to the amount of wound exudate, the presence of fibrin or necrotic tissue, and the depth of the wound. Hydrocolloids, hydrogels, chitin, polyurethane foams, alginates, and hydrofibers all have been recommended as treatment options for the local care of second-degree burn wounds [11]. Blisters that may be seen in superficial second-degree burns may serve as an excellent environment for the growth of microorganisms and increase the risk of infection. Small blisters may be left intact; however, large blisters should be removed, and the wound should be dressed [3, 12].

11.3.3. For deep second-degree, third-degree, and fourth-degree burns

The removal of the necrotic tissue, prevention of infection, and the maintenance of a moist environment are the primary goals to facilitate the wound healing in deep burns [11].

Eschar is the tough, leathery necrotic tissue seen in full-thickness burns. Circumferential eschar tissue may compromise circulation on extremities or restrict breathing over the chest. Escharotomy may be indicated in these patients. In the case of compartment syndrome, fasciotomy should be performed [3, 12]. Eschar tissue does not break down spontaneously, except in the case of infection [12]. Although the necrotic tissue of small deep burns may be treated by topical necrolytic agents, surgical debridement is needed in extensive burns [11]. As spontaneous healing is not expected and the scar formation is the final outcome of deep second-degree and third-degree burns, early excision of the eschar and grafting are the preferred treatments for these wounds. After the excision of eschar, temporary wound covering for the first days by topical antimicrobials (silver sulfadiazine) or wound dressings prevents infection and maintains moisture before surgery [1, 2, 11].

As the formation of scar can be prevented by the early and appropriate management of burn wound, excision should be done as soon as the patient is stabilized [3, 12]. Although the split-thickness autografts are the gold standard method in deep burns, they have many disadvantages. Allografts and xenografts may serve a good option for larger burns until the allografts are incorporated; however, they have also many limitations [1, 2]. Tissue engineering has provided a new era in the wound care field. Skin tissue regeneration by tissue-engineered products showed promising results in wound healing. Tissue scaffolds, healing-promoting factors (growth factors), stem cells, and gene therapy are the current solutions provided by bioengineering. Tissue scaffolds consist of epidermal, dermal, or composite substitutes which can provide a three-dimensional tissue for the optimal proliferation of cells and tissue regrowth. Several growth factors may be used as healing-promoting factors. Although the experimental studies with either embryonic or adult stem cells demonstrate the potential use of stem cells in the treatment of chronic wounds, further research is required to investigate their long-term effects on wound healing process. Gene therapy is a promising approach for the future treatment of burn wounds. It involves the transfer of genes into cells that encode growth factors required for enhancing wound repair. However, its use in burn wounds is limited by technical challenges. In conclusion, further trials are required to explore the long-term effects and safety of tissue engineering methods in burn wound treatment [1, 2, 24].

Fourth-degree burns are associated with significant functional impairments which require complicated and repeated surgeries. They often lead to amputations. Whereas local flaps may be used for the reconstruction of mild to moderate cases, burns with extensive damage need tissue transfers [1].

The common goal of all therapeutic tools abovementioned is to optimize wound healing, prevent scar formation, and minimize the functional disability. There are more other treatments that have been used for these purposes with varying success. Hyperbaric oxygen therapy has been suggested as a safe and effective treatment for burn wounds and can be used in conjunction with other modalities for burn patients [2, 25]. Silicone gels have been suggested to be useful in burns which carry high risk of hypertrophic scarring. They are recommended to be used before the maturation of scar [26]. Experimental studies showed promising results in the wound healing with platelet-rich plasma (PRP) treatment; however, its routine use in burn wounds and scars requires further evaluation [27]. Various types of lasers including pulse dye laser (PDL) and fractional ablative laser may offer better results when used in combination with surgery [28]. Pressure garments and massage therapy are also used to minimize scar contraction. Burn rehabilitation, splintage, and physiotherapy are very important to prevent contractures and to improve functional outcome. Additionally, as burn survivors may experience significant psychosocial problems, proper specialists should be consulted as soon as possible [3].

12. Malignancy on burn scars

Marjolin's ulcer is a rare cutaneous malignancy which may develop in burn scar. It occurs approximately two to three decades after the burn and is commonly seen on lower extremities as verrucous lesions. The squamous cell carcinoma is the most common form. The prevention of scar carcinoma by the early and effective treatment of scar formation is of primary importance to reduce the associated morbidity and mortality. Additionally, regular follow-up of patients with burn scars and early detection and evaluation of the non-healing ulcers are important considerations [29, 30].

Author details

Selda Pelin Kartal[1]*, Cemile Tuğba Altunel[2] and Dilek Bayramgurler[3]

*Address all correspondence to: pelin@dr.com

1 Dermatology Department, Diskapi Yildirim Beyazit Training and Research Hospital, University of Health Sciences, Ankara, Turkey

2 Dermatology Department, Private Natomed Hospital, Ankara, Turkey

3 Dermatology Department, Kocaeli University, Ankara, Turkey

References

[1] Oryan A, Alemzadeh E, Moshiri A. Burn wound healing: Present concepts, treatment strategies and future directions. Journal of Wound Care. 2017;**26**:5-19. DOI: 10.12968/jowc.2017.26.1.5

[2] Rowan MP, Cancio LC, Elster EA, Burmeister DM, Rose LF, Natesan S, Chan RK, Christy RJ, Chung KK. Burn wound healing and treatment: Review and advancements. Critical Care. 2015;**19**:243. DOI: 10.1186/s13054-015-0961-2

[3] Tiwari VK. Burn wound: How it differs from other wounds? Indian Journal of Plastic Surgery. 2012;**45**:364-373. DOI: 10.4103/0970-0358.101319

[4] Rybarczyk MM, Schafer JM, Elm CM, Sarvepalli S, Vaswani PA, Balhara KS, Carlson LC, Jacquet GA. Prevention of burn injuries in low- and middle-income countries: A systematic review. Burns. 2016;**42**:1183-1192. DOI: 10.1016/j.burns.2016.04.014

[5] Brusselaers N, Monstrey S, Vogelaers D, Hoste E, Blot S. Severe burn injury in Europe: A systematic review of the incidence, etiology, morbidity, and mortality. Critical Care. 2010; **14**:R188. DOI: 10.1186/cc9300

[6] Stylianou N, Buchan I, Dunn KW. A review of the international burn injury database (iBID) for England and Wales: Descriptive analysis of burn injuries 2003-2011. BMJ Open. 2015;**5**:e006184. DOI: 10.1136/bmjopen-2014-006184

[7] Golshan A, Patel C, Hyder AA. A systematic review of the epidemiology of unintentional burn injuries in South Asia. Journal of Public Health (Oxford, England). 2013;**35**:384-396. DOI: 10.1093/pubmed/fds102

[8] Veeravagu A, Yoon BC, Jiang B, Carvalho CM, Rincon F, Maltenfort M, Jallo J, Ratliff JK. National trends in burn and inhalation injury in burn patients: Results of analysis of the nationwide inpatient sample database. Journal of Burn Care & Research. 2015;**36**:258-265. DOI: 10.1097/BCR.0000000000000064

[9] Atiyeh BS, Costagliola M, Hayek SN. Burn prevention mechanisms and outcomes: Pitfalls, failures and successes. Burns. 2009;**35**:181-193. DOI: 10.1016/j.burns.2008.06.002

[10] Ansari-Moghaddam A, Baghbanian A, Dogoonchi M, Chooban B, Mostaghim-Roudi M, Torkfar G. Epidemiology of burn injuries in south-eastern Iran: A retrospective study. The Journal of the Pakistan Medical Association. 2013;**63**:1476-1481

[11] Yoshino Y, Ohtsuka M, Kawaguchi M, Sakai K, Hashimoto A, Hayashi M, et al. Wound/burn guidelines committee. The wound/burn guidelines-6: Guidelines for the management of burns. The Journal of Dermatology. 2016;**43**:989-1010. DOI: 10.1111/1346-8138.13288

[12] Yastı AÇ, Şenel E, Saydam M, Özok G, Çoruh A, Yorgancı K. Guideline and treatment algorithm for burn injuries. Ulusal Travma ve Acil Cerrahi Dergisi. 2015;**21**:79-89. DOI: 10.5505/tjtes.2015.88261

[13] Wibbenmeyer L, Liao J, Heard J, Kealey L, Kealey G, Oral R. Factors related to child maltreatment in children presenting with burn injuries. Journal of Burn Care & Research. 2014;**35**:374-381. DOI: 10.1097/BCR.0000000000000005

[14] Nielson CB, Duethman NC, Howard JM, Moncure M, Wood JG. Burns: Pathophysiology of systemic complications and current management. Journal of Burn Care & Research. 2017;**38**:e469-e481. DOI: 10.1097/BCR.0000000000000355

[15] Bittner EA, Shank E, Woodson L, Martyn JA. Acute and perioperative care of the burn-injured patient. Anesthesiology. 2015;**122**:448-464. DOI: 10.1097/ALN.0000000000000559

[16] Hettiaratchy S, Dziewulski P. ABC of burns: Pathophysiology and types of burns. British Medical Journal. Jun 12, 2004;**328**(7453):1427-1429

[17] Pham TN, Cancio LC, Gibran NS. American burn association practice guidelines burn shock resuscitation. Journal of Burn Care & Research. 2008;**29**:257-266

[18] Alencar de Castro RJ, Leal PC, Sakata RK. Pain management in burn patients. Brazilian Journal of Anesthesiology. 2013;**63**:149-153. DOI: 10.1016/S0034-7094(13)70206-X

[19] Tredget EE, Levi B, Donelan MB. Biology and principles of scar management and burn reconstruction. Surgical Clinics of North America. 2014;**94**:793-815. DOI: 10.1016/j.suc.2014.05.005

[20] Huang G, Liang B, Liu G, Liu K, Ding Z. Low dose of glucocorticoid decreases the incidence of complications in severely burned patients by attenuating systemic inflammation. Journal of Critical Care. 2015;**30**:436.e7-436.11. DOI: 10.1016/j.jcrc.2014.09.016

[21] Abdullahi A, Jeschke MG. Nutrition and anabolic pharmacotherapies in the care of burn patients. Nutrition in Clinical Practice. 2014;**29**:621-630

[22] Hahm G, Glaser JJ, Elster EA. Biomarkers to predict wound healing: The future of complex war wound management. Plastic and Reconstructive Surgery. 2011;**127**:21S-26S. DOI: 10.1097/PRS.0b013e3181fbe291

[23] Kaiser M, Yafi A, Cinat M, Choi B, Durkin AJ. Noninvasive assessment of burn wound severity using optical technology: A review of current and future modalities. Burns. 2011;**37**:377-386. DOI: 10.1016/j.burns.2010.11.012

[24] Shevchenko RV, James SL, James SE. A review of tissue-engineered skin bioconstructs available for skin reconstruction. Journal of The Royal Society Interface. 2010;**7**:229-258. DOI: 10.1098/rsif.2009.0403

[25] Cianci P, Slade JB Jr, Sato RM, Faulkner J. Adjunctive hyperbaric oxygen therapy in the treatment of thermal burns. Undersea & Hyperbaric Medicine. 2013;**40**:89-108

[26] Nedelec B, Carter A, Forbes L, Hsu SC, McMahon M, Parry I, et al. Practice guidelines for the application of nonsilicone or silicone gels and gel sheets after burn injury. Journal of Burn Care & Research. 2015;**36**:345-374. DOI: 10.1097/BCR.0000000000000124

[27] Ozcelik U, Ekici Y, Bircan HY, Aydogan C, Turkoglu S, Ozen O, Moray G, Haberal M. Effect of topical platelet-rich plasma on burn healing after partial-thickness burn injury. Medical Science Monitor. 2016;**22**:1903-1909

[28] Waibel J, Beer K. Ablative fractional laser resurfacing for the treatment of a third-degree burn. Journal of Drugs in Dermatology. 2009;**8**:294-297

[29] Das KK, Chakaraborty A, Rahman A, Khandkar S. Incidences of malignancy in chronic burn scar ulcers: Experience from Bangladesh. Burns. 2015;**41**:1315-1321. DOI: 10.1016/j.burns.2015.02.008

[30] Huang CY, Feng CH, Hsiao YC, Chuang SS, Yang JY. Burn scar carcinoma. The Journal of Dermatological Treatment. 2010;**21**:350-356. DOI: 10.3109/09546630903386580

Section 2

The Etiology, Pathophysiology and Clinical Findings of Burn Injury

Chapter 2

Burn Etiology and Pathogenesis

Yesim Akpinar Kara

Additional information is available at the end of the chapter

http://dx.doi.org/10.5772/intechopen.71379

Abstract

As a trauma type, "Burn" is one of the high-frequency accidents in the world. It is mostly caused by electricity, hot water, and chemical agents. A trauma can have acute effects on burns, skin, and other organ systems. These complications might be seen as myocardial infarction, thromboemboli, respiratory, and renal failure. In case of acute burns, the skin surface is severely destroyed. During this period, infection may develop on damaged skin. Therefore, in the treatment of burn wounds, protecting the damaged skin and multidisciplinary approaches are needed for preventing scar formation while healing process.

Keywords: burn etiology and pathophysiology, burn types, burn degrees, burn scar etiopathogenesis

1. Introduction

Burn is defined as destruction found in the epidermal tissue, dermal tissue, or deeper tissues, due to contact with thermal, chemical, or electrical agents. According to the World Health Organization, thermal burns account for an estimated 6.6 million injuries and 300,000 deaths each year worldwide [1]. Burn pathophysiology can be broken into local and systemic response. When excessive heat is transferred to the skin, it radiates outward from the point of initial contact and forms a local response with three zones in all directions. The systemic response following a burn can be massive. In a large burn, two clinically significant processes occur. The release of systemic inflammatory mediators and cytokines result in increased capillary permeability and wide scale extravasation of fluid and proteins from the intravascular to the extravascular space.

During wound healing, proinflammatory factors, such as interleukin (IL)-1, IL-6, and tumor necrosis factor-alpha (TNF-alpha) are released. This promote chronic inflammation and various inflammatory cells are formed in the affected tissue. Angiogenesis starts into the damaged tissue. Tumor necrosis factor-alpha, prostaglandin E2 also play a role in the formation of inflammatory response in wound healing. Any damage to the formation of this response can result in scarring after the burn. The primary cytokine responsible for scar formation is transforming growth factor-beta (TGF-β) secretion which is released from the other inflammatory cells and myofibroblasts. Hypertrophic scar does not develop when the reticular layer is not affected in burning. As a result, inflammatory cells, fibroblasts, newly formed blood vessels, and collagen deposits develop hypertrophic scar tissue in the reticular layer [2, 3].

2. Description

The skin, which is the largest organ of the body, constitutes 16% of the total body weight. It is 6–10 kg and 1.5–2 m^2 in length in adult man. The skin is a protective covering for the organism and also acts as a sensory organ. It regulates body temperature and blood pressure by means of dermal vascular component. It synthesizes vitamin D3 with the effect of ultraviolet. Stratum corneum creates a barrier to prevent fluid and electrolyte loss and regulates transepidermal fluid passage. It provides homeostasis of the body against trauma that can be caused by various physical and chemical factors originating from the external environment [4]. Physical and chemical agents cause various damages to be formed directly, with thermal, mechanical, and radial factors, or as a result of the reactions they create [4].

Dermatitis developed due to high temperature trauma is defined as burn. Burn is an acute tissue injury caused by exposure to materials, solid or liquid, hot or showing effects of hot [5]. In skin and/or subcutaneous tissues, all of the acute damage caused by exposure to heat, cold, electricity, radiation, or chemical agents is burn. Although the developed damage is in the skin and subcutaneous tissues, it is a very comprehensive trauma that affects the entire organism due to the conditions, such as the depth of the burn, the surface area, the causative agent, and the infection and metabolic circumstances that may occur in the follow-up process, that determines the prognosis with the pathophysiology it caused [5, 6]. The skin loses its functions when it is burned. Burns can spread from outer layers of skin to deeper tissues [5].

The form of occurrence and duration of exposure to the active agent (flame, liquid, gas, chemical agents, etc.) is important in planning the treatment. A more detailed evaluation of the patient should be examined about general examination findings accompanying the burn. Whether there is evidence of dry cough, hoarseness, and breathing difficulties suggesting inhalation injury should be questioned in burns that develop due to flames. The anamnesis of the burn plays an important role, especially since antidote treatment may be needed aimed to the agent in chemical burns.

3. History

The first written documents about burns were found 2400 years ago during the times of Hippocrates. In 1607, Hildanus had graded the burns. In 1799, Earle found that applying ice water to the burned area could prevent pain. During World War I, burns related to the use of sulfur-containing chemicals were observed and advanced treatment facilities were established for the treatment of burns after World War II [7].

4. Epidemiology

Although the awareness level of the individuals is increasing nowadays and preventive technologies are developed, the burn is still one of the important causes of mortality and high morbidity. It is known that more than 6 million people are exposed to burns every year in the world, and that the mortality rate due to burns is 6–7%. About 75% of the deaths are due to CO inhalation and at the scene primarily [8]. Another cause of mortality is sepsis. As the total body surface area affected by burn increases, the mortality rate also increases [8]. Burns are most commonly seen in the upper and lower extremities [8, 9]. Burn traumas often result from an accident or neglect. About 80% of the burns arise from individual errors and 70% occur at home [4]. Burn epidemiology varies with age. Child age group and elderly population are more at risk. Studies show that more than half of the cases are in the child age group. About 19% are under the age of 5 and 12% are over 60 years old [1]. While boiled water and flame burns are seen most commonly, they are followed by electrical and chemical burns. While hot water burns are seen in approximately 70% of the pediatric age group, burns due to flame at home or office are seen in adults [10]. In a study conducted in Tokyo, 82% of cases were due to hot water and 11% of cases were due to flames in children under 16 years of age [11]. In the study of Aytaç et al. causes of burns were found as 68.8% hot water, 1.5% flame, 3.8% hot material contact injuries, and 1.1% chemical burns, respectively [9].

5. Etiology

At least 44°C of heat is required for the skin to be burned. Besides, the duration of the heat is also important; transepidermal necrosis occurring with 70°C of heat in a second, occurs in 45 minutes with 47°C of heat [4].

Burns can be grouped according to thermal, chemical, electricity, and radiation [12]. The causative of burns should be known since a different treatment protocol is applied in each case. Thermal burns that occur with direct effects of flames with high levels of heat, contact with hot objects, hot liquids, or hot vapors are commonly seen. The duration of the contact and the degree of the temperature determine the degree of cell damage [1]. Chemical burns due to acid or alkali salts and solutions may cause burns due to corrosive effects of these substances. Other than these, burns can also develop due to electrical current, radiation, ultraviolet, and laser rays [4]. Serious burns due to flames of weapons, explosives, and combustibles can occur during warfare [12].

5.1. Thermal burns

It develops in two different ways as hot water and flame burns. Thermal burns are skin injuries caused by excessive heat, typically from contact with hot surfaces, hot liquids, steam, or flame. Thermal damage to skin results in cellular death as a function of temperature and length of contact time. Thermal burns are the most common type of burn injuries, making up about 86% of the burned patients requiring burn center admission. About 70% of the burns in children develop due to hot water. It is most often caused by hot drinks or hot bath water. These burns are usually first-degree or superficial second-degree burns [13, 14]. Flame burns account for 50% of adult burns [14]. Inhalation burn may also develop together with it. It usually appears as a second or third-degree burn.

5.2. Chemical burns

It is the cause of burns caused by cleaning materials that are used in daily life at home or by work accidents. While 3–6% of all burns constitute chemical burns, they constitute 14–30% of burn-related mortalities [15]. Generally, it is developed due to contact with strong acid or alkaline substances. Unlike thermal burns, there is longer contact with the agent. Inhalation or ingestion of the chemical material may result in systemic symptoms and injuries in the mouth, esophagus, and stomach where it contacts. Bleach, cement, plaster, and hydrofluoric acid used in glassware artwork, phenol, and petroleum-derived organic compounds, phosphorus used in the construction of various warfare materials are the most common reasons of chemical burn incidents [12].

Acid burns tend to limit themselves. Hydrofluoric acid is one of the most frequently used acids for construction of electrical circuits and for scraping paintings on glass and that causes burn most [16]. Hydrofluoric acid passes quickly through the skin and continues to damage tissue until it reaches a tissue rich in calcium, such as bone. Even small hydrofluoric acid burns may develop hypocalcemia, which is sufficient for cardiac effects to occur. More than 10% hydrofluoric acid may be fatal. The gels containing calcium gluconate can be administered topically, or IV calcium gluconate can be given in severe cases [16].

Bleach, oven cleaners, fertilizer, cement, plaster, and lime contact result in basic burns. Bases penetrate deep into the tissue, combine with cutaneous lipids to form soap, and continue to dissolve the skin until neutralized. Pain in the base burns occurs late, which delays first aid. Base burns are more dangerous than acid burns [16].

Phenol and petroleum-derived compounds are organic compounds. They break down proteins by direct reactions or production of heat [14].

Compounds containing sodium, phosphorus, lithium, and chlorine are inorganic compounds. They cause skin damage by direct bonding and salt formation [14].

Some modern bombs contain white phosphorus. When this element comes into contact with air, it burns and the oil-soluble phosphorus fragments are scattered across the wound and spread through the subcutaneous fat tissue. As long as phosphorus is in contact with oxygen, it continues to burn, and therefore phosphorus burns are deep and painful, may extend to the bone. Local treatment is more urgent than conventional burns. Phosphorus burns must be prevented from contacting with air; it should be isolated by wrapping the wound with wet dressings or by immersing the affected areas in water. It should not be allowed to remain dry at any times. Phosphorus can cause hypocalcemia and hyperphosphatemia. There may be many unwanted effects of absorbed phosphorus, delirium, psychosis, convulsions, coma; hepatomegaly, jaundice; proteinuria, acute tubular necrosis; thrombocytopenia, hypoprothrombinemia, ventricular arrhythmia, and myocarditis may develop [4, 14].

Other than these, burns due to coal tar can also develop, especially in the treatment of psoriasis. Tar is an industrial material used in road cladding and roof isolation [17]. It is obtained by dry distillation from organic substances, has a liquid oil consistency and is a water-insoluble substance. The boiling point reaches up to 232°C. This may cause severe burns. In the literature, it has been shown that the majority of hot tar burns often occur in the workplace in male workers with accidents [18]. Continuation of the skin contact with tar causes the heat transfer to continue and leads the burn to progress. Therefore, the tar should be removed from the body in a short time. In the literature, successful cases have been reported in which unsterilized sunflower oil, olive oil, as well as lanolin and surfactant-containing creams and other antibiotic creams were used [19]. Again, in the tar adhered skin zone, the ice cubes were left for 10–20 minutes, and the tar was frozen and separated in the form of a crust.

Chemical burns due to mercury-containing substances can cause blistering (bullae). Blisters must be excised because mercury is found in the bullae liquid.

5.3. Electrical burns

Electric burns, which are most common in men between 20 and 40 years of age, constitute 20% of burn-related mortalities [15]. It occurs by electric current or lightning strike. Low-voltage electrical burns are considered to be less than 1000 volts and high-voltage electrical burns are considered to be more than 1000 volts; electrical burns between 250 and 1000 volts should be followed up just like high-voltage electrical burns since these patients may develop unconsciousness, compartment syndrome, and myoglobinuria/hemoglobinuria [15].

In low-voltage accidents, burns are limited on the skin, however, go down into deeper tissues. In high-voltage accidents, there are traces just like stapler pierce, ulceration, and scarring. In the lightning strike, necrotic areas start from where the current entered and progress along the line [4]. As a result of direct contact with the electricity, systemic complications such as cardiac arrhythmia, necrotic areas in the soft tissues and bones may develop as well as thermal damage as the current passes through the whole body.

5.4. Radiation burns

It is caused by the uptake of radioactive material. The local radiation burns caused by high radiation doses (8–10 Gy) are similar to thermal burns except for several days to weeks of delayed latency. Taking high doses causes sudden cell death. The most sensitive tissues to radiation are lymphocytes and hematopoietic cells. The degree of radiation damage depends on the dose [20]. Erythema on the skin is the earliest finding. After weeks of exposure to high-dose radiation, necrosis and ulceration of the skin may develop.

Although it is not dependent on excessive heat or flame, sunburns and frostbites should be considered in the integrity of the burn etiology.

5.5. Sunburns

It develops due to uncontrolled and prolonged exposure to sun or light sources containing UVB. Sunburn is the contact dermatitis due to ultraviolet B rays (295–315 nm), which is the most erythematous wavelength. The formation of sunburn requires more ultraviolet light than the minimal erythematous dose (MED) [10]. While 20 minutes is enough to get a minimal erythematous dose (MED) in a clear summer day, 1 full day sunbathing is needed to reach 20 times the MED dose. People reaching this dose have sunburns with individual differences. The skin reaction starts at 4–6 hours and ends at 72 hours [4].

5.6. Cold burn (frostbite)

It is developed with cooling of the body. The skin is frozen at −2 to −10°C and irreversible changes occur under −22°C. Cold burn is different from thermal burns; trauma occurs at the cellular level and extracellular fluid directly, at the organ functions indirectly [21]. Electrolyte concentration increases with development of ice crystals in the intracellular and extracellular fluid, enzyme systems do not work and tissue destruction begins [4]. Vasoconstriction endothelial damage and thromboembolism increases ischemia and failure [21]. Prostoglandins are primarily responsible cytokines. In the first-degree frostbite, firstly, reflex erythema starts against cold, then vasoconstruction and paleness are seen. In the second-degree frostbite, erythema, edema, and subepidermal bullae, in the third-degree frostbite, blue-black color changes and hardening are observed [4]. It is usually seen at the outer regions such as ear, nose, and fingers [10]. Ischemia developed in the tissue and is spread to the body.

Besides these burn types, other rare burn traumas have been reported. There are also types of burns that are common in eastern societies and are associated with low socio-cultural level. As an alternative to modern medicine, particularly those commonly used in muscle joint disorders, include herbal applications and cupping therapy [22].

6. Physiopathology

6.1. Local and systemic changes in the formation of burn scars

When burns occur, cell proteins in the skin denature and coagulate and thrombosis develops in the vessels. Vascular permeability increases and denatured cell particles increase intercellular osmotic pressure. Vasoactive amines such as histamine, kinin, prostaglandin, and serotonin are released from the burn developing tissue. Platelet and leukocyte adhesion to endothelium occurs. The complement system is activated cytotoxic T cells increase, and the tissue develops into an open site for infection [23].

Heat injuries occur in two stages. First, coagulative type necrosis develops in the epidermis and tissues. Afterwards, late type injury occurs due to cell lysis as a result of progression of dermal ischemia (within 24–48 hours). The depth of necrosis is determined by degree of temperature it is exposed to and the time of duration [24].

Burn injury causes both local and systemic changes. Vasodilatation and vascular permeability are also increased in the skin and subcutaneous tissues due to local reaction. As a systemic response, all internal organ systems are affected **(Figure 1).** In severe burns, cytokines and other inflammatory mediators are released in excess both in the burn area and in the unburned areas. These mediators cause vasoconstriction and vasodilatation, increase in capillary permeability, and development of edema both in the burn site and in remote organs. Pathological changes occur in metabolic, cardiovascular, renal, gastrointestinal, and coagulation systems. With burn shock, blood volume and cardiac output are decreased, renal blood flow and glomerular filtration rate decrease, gastrointestinal mucosal atrophy develops and intestinal permeability increases. Catabolism is accelerated and often results in widespread microthrombosis [14, 25].

When the burn occurs, three damage zones are described as local changes in the skin. These regions were first described by Jackson in 1947 [13]. It consists of coagulation (necrosis) zone, stasis (ischemia) zone and the outermost hyperthermia (inflammation) zone (**Figure 2**). The innermost region is the area closest to the heat source and the one with the greatest damage. Coagulation of structural proteins that develop in this region results in irreversible tissue injury. The area outside this region is called the stasis (ischemic) zone. In this area, tissue perfusion has reduced but is a layer of living tissue. Cells in this area can be saved if treatment is done to increase tissue perfusion. Otherwise, progressive ischemia and necrosis develop within 24–48 hours [13]. The third and outermost zone is hyperemia (inflammation) zone. Tissue perfusion is increased in this region and is characterized by vasodilation due to the

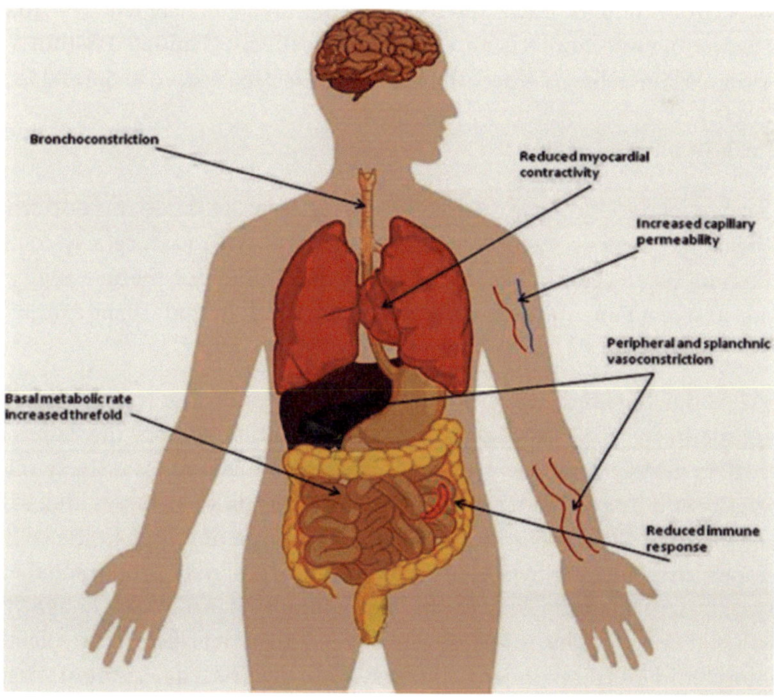

Figure 1. Systemic changes that occur after a burn injury.

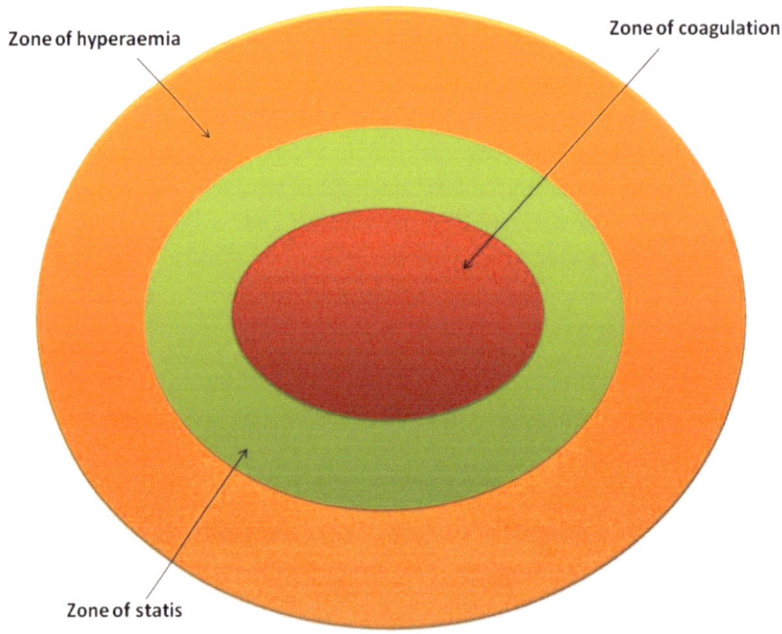

Figure 2. Jackson's burns zones.

inflammation surrounding the burn. The tissues in this area will heal within 7–10 days unless there is an intervening infection. It is important that treatment is initiated within 24 hours due to necrosis progression in burns where the stasis zone is progressive to dermal ischemia [26].

6.2. Burn shock ve pathogenesis

If the burn area exceeds 30% of the total body surface area, cytokines released from the burn area and other inflammatory mediators reach levels that will produce a systemic response [13]. An inflammatory reaction also occurs as a result of a minor thermal injury lasting for 20–60 seconds and at a temperature of 51–60°C. Burn shock period can be examined in three periods:

Early period (exudative period): It covers the first 36–72 hours after trauma. Vasodilatation is the first response to trauma in the burn area. Systemic inflammatory mediators (histamine, TNF-α, IL-1, IL-6, GM-CSF, interferon-ɤ, and prostaglandins) are excessively released from both the burn site and from other tissues. Capillary permeability increases, due to inadequate tissue perfusion, intracellular sodium increases, and edema develops in the cells [27]. Burn shock developed after burns is hypovolemic shock and is directly proportional to the extent and severity of burns. In adults 20%, in children younger than 12 years of age 10%, of burn area leads to a higher risk for hypovolemic shock development [4, 24]. Hypovolemia resulting from circulatory fluid loss due to edema, occurs within the first 2 days utmost. Hemodynamic insufficiency develops due to decreased blood volume. As circulation in the brain, kidneys, liver, muscles, and gastrointestinal system deteriorates, oxygenation is reduced. Ischemia develops in the tissues as a result of hypovolemia and slowing down of blood flow. Damage to cells that develops in hypoxia leads to dysfunction in organs [13, 24]. Clinical signs of hypovolemic shock are observed as follows:

- Pale, moist, cool skin.
- Hyperthermia have coldness at extremities.
- Tachycardia and hypotension.
- Fast and shallow breathing.
- Decrease in urine volume.

Intermediate period (intoxication period): Includes 2–4 weeks after burn. During this period, the formation of edema stops and polyuria develops. While edema is regressing, the denatured proteins released from the cells pass through the circulation to form the intoxication case. At the end of the first week after burn, the hemodynamic situation is completely reversed and there is an abnormally high cardiac output accompanied by vasodilatation in the burn patient. On the 10th day after the burn, the cardiac output is increased by 2.5 times of normal [28].

Late (infectious) period: Acute and chronic infections may occur during this period. The cellular and humoral immune response is suppressed in direct proportion to the size of the burn. Lymphopenia develops chemotaxis, phagocytosis, and migration of neutrophils are reduced. IL-2 level decreases in burns that hold large surface area. IL-1, IL-6, and IL-8 levels decrease in the first week after burn [23]. Increased catabolism and capillary leakage result in reduced circulating IgG, IgA, and IgM. The decrease in IgG, especially after burn injuries, is closely related to septic complications [13, 29]. With respect to the grade of the burn, T cell activation is impaired, creating a predisposing condition for viral and fungal infections [24].

6.3. Evaluation of burn severity

The determination of the severity of a burn depends on the depth of the burn and the width of the area. It is necessary to wait 24–48 hours to determine the exact burn grade, as the depth of the burn may increase due to edema and infection [4, 10].

The depth of the burn varies according to the type of the causative agent, the degree of temperature, and the thickness and vascularity of the affected skin area. Burn depth is examined in three groups **(Figure 3)**.

- First-degree burn is a superficial burn and there is only damage in epidermis. There is a painful erythema and edema in the burned skin. Pain relieves after 12–24 hours, first-degree burn heals with desquamation 1 week later; does not leave any cicatrix. Sunburns are considered as first-degree burns. Cold application to erythematous and edematous area also reduces pain. Topical analgesic creams can be applied as symptomatic treatment [28].
- Second-degree burn occurs in two forms: superficial and deep. The epidermis and the dermis layer down to the sebaceous glands are affected in the superficial type [4]. Edema

and subepidermal bullae formation are observed on the skin. Hair roots are intact and not affected by burns. In the deep type, burn goes down as far as to reticular dermis. The skin is pale and thickened. Some areas have erythema, if the bullae are opened, the surface appears moist due to plasma leak. If the skin surface remains dry during this period, the pain will increase, so wet dressing should be done. A superficial type of second-degree burn heals within 2–4 weeks without cicatrix. Hypo-hyperpigmentation may develop. In the deep type, healing is slow, may exceed to 4 weeks, and healing results in cicatrix. There may be loss of function in skin and hair. Fluid resuscitation may be needed for second-degree burns that hold more than 20% of the total body surface area [28, 30].

- Whole skin (epidermis, dermis, and hypodermis) is affected in third-degree burns. More severe burns can affect muscles, tendons, and bones. The skin surface is dry and free from erythema. This tissue, which has lost its vitality and is hard, is defined as eschar. A few days later, when the eschar layer is removed, deep granulation tissue is observed. This tissue absolutely heals with cicatrix. Large scars do not close up and skin grafting may be necessary [31].

Accurate calculation of the burn surface area, as well as burn depth, is very important for the initiation of emergency treatment and fluid replacement. When the surface area of the burn is determined, what percentage of the whole body surface area is burned is calculated. The body surface area of a normal adult is about 1.72 m^2 [4, 10]. "Rule of Nines" of Wallace is used to determine the area of the burned surface **(Figure 4)**. With this approach, the burned area is calculated approximately in a short time.

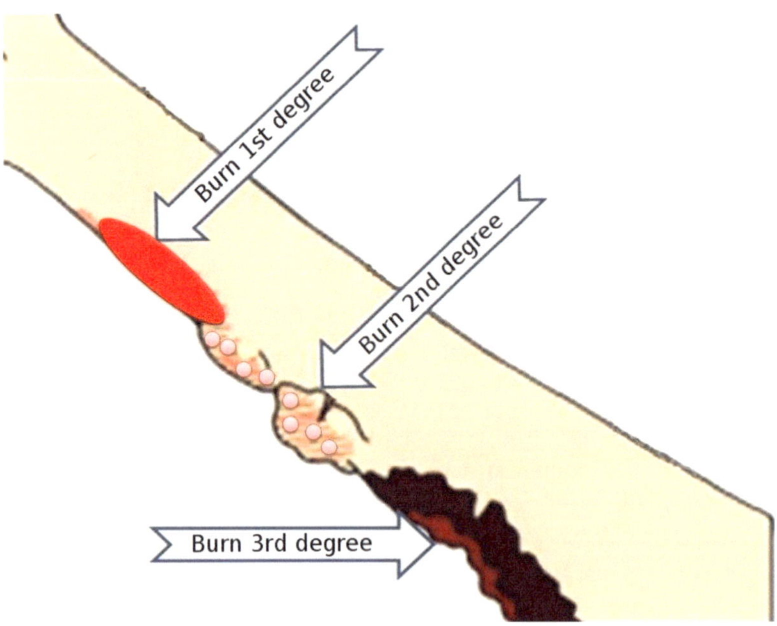

Figure 3. Burn types.

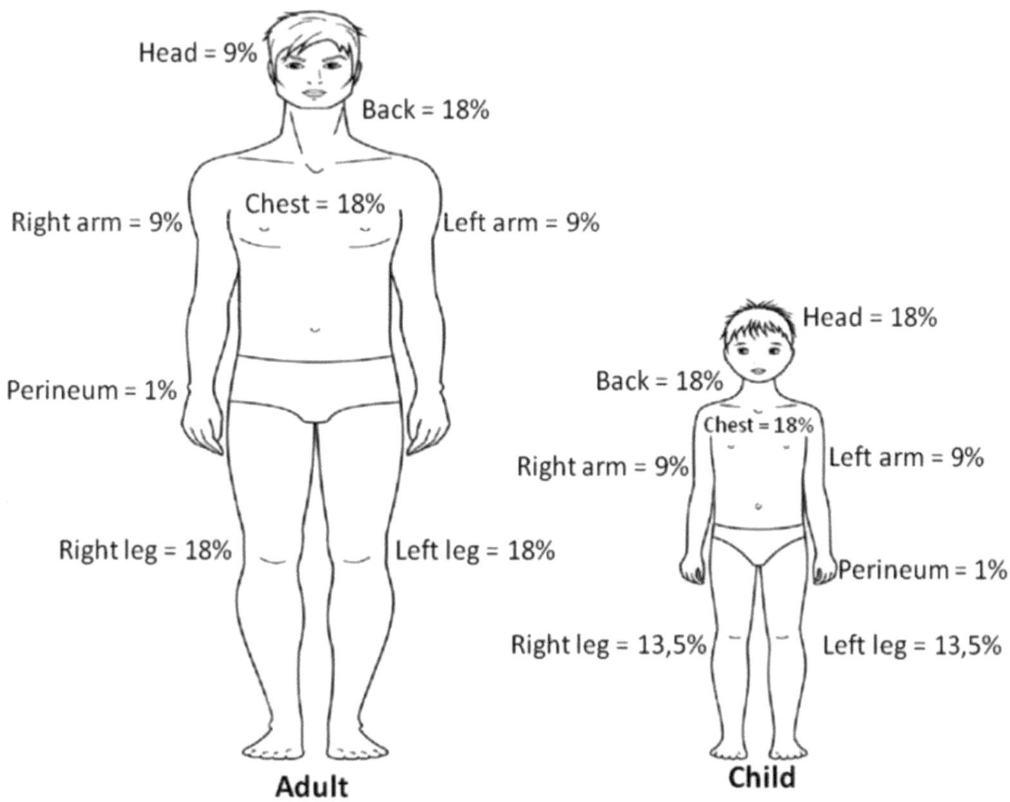

Figure 4. Wallas rule of nines.

According to the Rule of Nines, head is 9%, each upper limb is 9%, each lower limb is 18%, anterior trunk except head and extremities is 18%, posterior trunk is 18%, and perineal region is 1% of total body surface area. The palm area of a patient, including the fingers, constitutes 0.8% of the total body surface area. The palmar surface area is generally used to estimate small or large burns [32]. In children, the head and neck region has a larger portion of the entire body surface. The lower limbs form smaller body surface area. Because of this, Rule of Nines can not be applied to children under 14 years old. Therefore "Lund and Browder Chart" has been developed (**Figure 5**).

Burns with area smaller than 5% are considered as simple burns. About 1–15% burn in adults (1–7% in children) is "mild burn", above 15% deep burn in adults (7% in children) is "severe burn" and 40% superficial burn in adults (20% in children) is "intermediate burn", above 30% deep burn in adults (20% in children) "severe burn" involving the face and upper respiratory tract and severe electrical burns. There is a high risk of developing hypovolemic shock in second- and third-degree burns with 10% area in children and elderly, and with 15% area in other age groups [32].

Pigmented skin may be difficult to evaluate, in such cases it may be necessary to remove all loose epidermal layers to calculate the extent of burn [48].

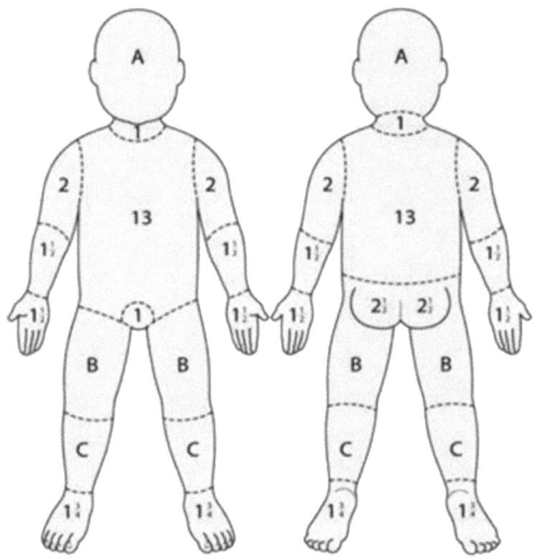

Area	Age 0	1	5	10	15	Adult
A= ½ of head	9½	8½	6½	5½	4½	3½
B=½ of one thigh	2¾	3¼	4	4½	4½	4¾
C= ½ of one lower leg	2½	2½	2¾	3	3¼	3½

Figure 5. Lund and browder chart.

7. Burn scars

It is estimated that more than 6 million people per year have burn wounds. Despite improvements in treatment and survival rates, scar formation rates are high and such scars cause severe functional impairment, psychological morbidity, and costly long-term treatments [33].

Scars that develop are often late complications of the burn, usually seen after an inadequate and inappropriate treatment for burn wounds as well as immediately after the treatment. Post-burn cicatrix can be divided into three main groups: hypertrophic, atrophic scars, and contractures [34]. In a study conducted in Italy, in cases 23 days after reepithelialization and meanly 15 months after; hypertrophic scars in 77%, contracture in 44%, hypertrophic contracture scars in 5%, hypertrophic induction in 28% were observed to be developed [33]. Especially hypertrophic scars that develop after thermal injuries may be together with contracture, which can also lead to loss of function in joints [34, 35].

Burn wound healing occurs in three phases. These are the inflammation, proliferation, and remodeling phases. Prolongation and expansion of the inflammatory phase is the most important factor in scar formation [36]. Scar formation is affected by the depth of the burn, the duration of the healing, the development of infection, the age of the patient, genetic factors, circulatory disturbances, or the development of diseases that suppress the immune system [37].

In particular, hypertrophic scars or keloids do not develop in burns that do not reach reticular dermis. During wound healing, several factors increase or prolong the inflammation in the reticular dermis. In a study conducted, the most frequent factors in scar development were found to be flame-induced burns, followed by hot water and less frequently as chemical and electrical burns [34]. The development of infection or folliculitis in the wound bed, mechanical trauma, large and deep burns, and improper treatment in the first period increase the risk of scar development [38]. The rate of hypertrophic scar development in burns recovered under 10 days is 4%, while the risk of scar development in burn wounds healing in 21 days or longer is up to 70% [39]. One of the most important factors in pathological wound healing is mechanical stretching of the skin [45, 46, 48]. Anterior chest wall, arms, and shoulders are the most common areas for hypertrophic scars. Another risk factor for scar development is that the person is adolescent or pregnant. Vasodilator effects of hormones such as estrogen and androgens increase scar development. Children and adolescents with pigmentation injury skin type were more likely to develop scarring [40, 41]. In a study by Arima and colleagues, hypertension was found to be another risk factor for the development of scarring [42]. Among burn cases with systemic inflammation, the patients who undergo reconstructive surgery have been shown to develop scarring within 1 year [38]. Predisposing factors for scar development include A blood group, hyperimmunoglobulin E syndrome (high allergy risk), Afro-American, and Asian ethnicity [43]. Wound healing is a natural process that reinstates deep integrity of the skin as quickly as possible. Wound healing can lead to an excessive process that is causing pathological scar formation or to a dynamic process that does not heal or turns into a chronic wound. Singer and Clark argue that hypertrophic scar formation is caused by an abnormal wound healing [35]. Unlike keloids, the hypertrophic wound remains at its limits and these marks can regress over time [44].

7.1. Pathophysiology

TGF-β is the most important cytokine involved in wound healing. TGF-β plays a role in fibroblast proliferation, collagen synthesis, and storage and reshaping of the new extracellular matrix (ECM) by stimulating inflammation and angiogenesis [45]. It has been demonstrated by several groups that fibroblasts derived from hypertrophic scarring have a phenotype that varies from normal scars or fibroblasts produced from undamaged dermis [2]. Wang et al. have shown that hypertrophic fibroblasts and hypertrophic scar tissue produce more mRNA and protein for TGF-β1 compared to normal skin-derived normal skin or fibroblasts, suggesting that TGF-β1 may play a role in hypertrophic scar formation [3]. Type 1 and type 2 collagen synthesis is increased by smooth muscle expression with proliferation in myofibroblasts, which leads to fibrosis.

In hypertrophic scars, it has been shown that type III collagen fibers which are parallel to the epidermal surface predominate. Scar tissue consists mainly of differentiated fibroblast nodules including myofibroblasts, collagen filaments, and other extracellular matrix proteins [2]. Immediately after injury, platelet degranulation and activation of the complement and coagulation stages occur. For hemostasis, fibrin clots form and become a framework for wound repair [2]. Together with platelet degranulation, a number of potent cytokines such as epidermal growth factor (EGF), insulin growth factor (IGF-I), platelet-derived growth factor (PDGF), and transforming growth factor (TGF-β1) are released. Fibroblasts synthesize the reparative tissue skeleton, called the extracellular matrix (ECM). This granulation tissue consists of procollagen, elastin, proteoglycans, and hyaluronic acid. Decorin, a proteoglycan, is found extensively in the dermal extracellular matrix. Decorin regulates collagen fibril, fiber, and fiber bundle organization, and has been shown to reduce approximately 75% in hypertrophic scars [3]. Decorin can bind to TGF-β and neutralize it, thus minimizing the stimulatory effects of this cytokine on collagen, fibronectin, and glycosaminoglycan production. The conversion of a wound clot to granulation tissue requires a precise balance between ECM protein accumulation and disintegration, and when this procedure is impaired, scarring abnormalities occur [46].

As mediators of the TGF-β pathway, SMADs are the intracellular protein family that regulates the signaling of the TGF-β type I receptor in response of the cell to a specific TGF-β. R-SMAD3 and 4 were identified as predominant mediators of autocrine stimulation with TGF-β in hypertrophic wound-derived fibroblasts [46].

Other than these, keratinocytes are thought to play an important role in scar formation by producing signals that stimulate fibroblasts in the dermis or by producing more ECM [47, 48]. It has been shown that the mast cells that mediate the secretion of soluble mediators such as histamine, heparin, and cytokines promote fibroblast proliferation [47].

In particular, IL-1β, PDGF, EGF, and TNF-α play an important role in the expression of matrix metalloprotein in fibroblasts and are responsible for scar formation [49, 50]. Apoptosis has also been shown to play a critical role in the transition to scar formation following tissue damage [47, 50].

Author details

Yesim Akpinar Kara

Address all correspondence to: yesim_akpinar@yahoo.com

Department of Dermatology, Ufuk University, Ankara, Turkey

References

[1] American Burn Association. Burn Incidence and Treatment in the United States. 2016. Available from: http://www.ameriburn.org/resources_factsheet.php [Accessed: June 22, 2016]

[2] Ali SS, Hajrah NH, Ayuob NN, Moshref SS, Abuzinadah OA. Morphological and morphometric study of cultured fibroblast from treated and untreated abnormal scar. Saudi Medical Journal. 2010;**30**:874-881

[3] Scott PG et al. Chemical characterization and quantification of proteoglycans in human post-burn hypertrophic and mature scars. Clinical Science (London, England). 1996; **90**:417-425

[4] Keck M, Herndon DH, Kamolz LP, Frey M, Jeschke MG. Pathophysiology of burns. Wiener Medizinische Wochenschrift. 2009;**159**(13-14):327-336

[5] Rao K, Ali SN, Moiemen NS. Etiology and outcome of burns in the elderly. Burns. Nov 2006;**32**(7):802-805

[6] Gianfaldoni R, Gianfaldoni S, Lotti J, Tchernev G, Wollina U, Lotti T. The importance of first aid to burned patients: 30 Years of experience at the burns Centre in Pisa. Macedonian Journal of Medical Sciences. Jul 23, 2017;**5**(4):420-422

[7] Sibel ÖG, Tayfun Y. Yanık giriş,epidemiyoloji ve etyolojisi. Turkiye Klinikleri Journal of Medical Sciences. 2007;**3**(1):1-3

[8] Pham TN, Cancio LC, Gibran NS. American burn association practice guidelines burn shock resuscitation. Journal of Burn Care & Research. 2008;**29**:257-266

[9] Brusselaers N, Monstrey S, Vogelaers D, Hoste E, Blot S. Severe burn injury in Europe: A systematic review of the incidence, etiology, morbidity, and mortality. Critical Care. 2010;**14**:R188

[10] Freedberg IM, Eısen AZ, Wolf K, Austen KF, Goldsmith L, Katz S, Fitzpatrick TB. Dermatology in General Medicine. 5th ed. p. 1505-1513

[11] Kobayashi K, Ikedal H, Higuchi R, Nozaki M, et al. Epidemiological and outcome characteristics of major burns in Tokyo. Burns. 2005;**31**(1):3-11

[12] Ramponi DR. Chemical burns of the eye. Advanced Emergency Nursing Journal. Jul/Sep 2017;**39**(3):193-198

[13] Yin S. Chemical and common burns in children. Clinical Pediatrics (Phila). May 2017;**56** (5 Suppl):8S-12S

[14] Hettiaratchy S, Dziewulski PABC. Of burns: Pathophysiology and types of burns. British Medical Journal. Jun 12, 2004;**328**:1427-1429

[15] Foris LA, Huecker MR. Electrical Injuries. StatPearls [Internet]. Treasure Island (FL): StatPearls Publishing; Jun–Aug 21, 2017

[16] Kirkpatrick JJ, Enion DS, Burd DA. Hydrofluoric acid burns: A review. Burns. 1995;**21**:483-493

[17] Ersel M, Aksay E, Özsaraç M, Yüksel B. Use of olive oil for clening of hot tar burn. Turkish Journal of Emergency Medicine. 2009;**9**(4):174-176

[18] Robinett DA, Shelton B, Dyer KS. Special consideration in hazardous materials burns. Journal of Emergency Medicine. Apr 8, 2008 e-pub

[19] Levy DB, Barone JA, York JM, Raia JJ. Unibase and triple antibiotic ointment for hardened tar removal. Annals of Emergency Medicine. 1986;**15**(6):765-766

[20] Lee JO, Herndon DN. Burns and radiation injuries. In: Feliciano DV, Kenneth L, Moore EE, editors. Trauma. 6th ed. McGraw-Hill; 2008. p. 1051-1066

[21] Nizamoglu M, Tan A, Vickers T, Segaren N, barnes D, Dziewulski P. Cold burn injuries in the UK: The 11-year experience of a tertiary burns centre. Burns & Trauma. Nov 11, 2016;**4**:36

[22] Akbulut S, Semur H, Köse O, Ozhasenekler A, Celiktas M, Basbug M, Yagmur Y. Phytocontact dermatitis due to *Ranunculus arvensis* mimicking burn injury: Report of three cases and literature review. International Journal of Emergency Medicine. 2011;**4**:7

[23] Rae L, Fidler P, Gibran N. The physiologic basis of burn shock and the need for aggressive fluid resuscitation. Critical Care Clinics. Oct 2016;**32**(4):491-505

[24] Singh V, Devgan L, Bhat S, Milner SM. The pathogenesis of burn wound conversion. Annals of Plastic Surgery. 2007;**59**(1):109-115

[25] Lund T, Onarheim H, Reed RK. Pathogenesis of edema formation in burn injuries. World Journal of Surgery. 1992;**16**(1):2-9

[26] Gueugniaud PY, Carsin H, Bertin-Maghit M, Petit P. Current advances in the initial management of major thermal burns. Critical Care Medicine. 2000;**26**:848-856

[27] Demling RH. The burn edema process:Current concepts. The Journal of Burn Care & Rehabilitation. 2005;**26**(3):207-227

[28] Martin NA, Falder S. A review of the evidence for threshold of burn injury. Burns. May 20, 2017. pii: S0305-4179(17)30215-2

[29] Rose T, Verbeken G, Vos DD, Merabishvili M, Vaneechoutte M, Lavigne R, Jennes S, Zizi M, Pirnay JP. Experimental phage therapy of burn wound infection: Difficult first steps. International Journal of Burns and Trauma. Oct 26, 2014;**4**(2):66-73

[30] Pavoni V, Gianesello L, Paparella L, Buoninsegni LT, Barboni E. Outcome predictors and quality of life of severe burn patients admitted to intensisve care unit. Scandinavian Journal of Trauma, Resuscitation and Emergency Medicine. 2010;**27**(18):24

[31] Kao CC, Garner WL. Acute burns. Plastic and Reconstructive Surgery. 2000;**105**:2482-2493

[32] Hettiaratchy S, Papini R. Initial management of a major burn: II-Assessment and resuscitation. British Medical Journal. Jul 10, 2004;**329**:101-103

[33] Taal L, Faber AW. Posttraumatic stress and maladjustment among adult burn survivors 1 to 2 years post burn. Part III. The interview data. Burns. 1998;**24**:399-405

[34] Gangemi EN, Gregori D, Berchialla P, Zingarelli E, Cairo M, Bollero D, Ganem J, Capocelli R, Cuccuru F, Cassano P, Risso D, Stella M. Epidemiology and risk factors for pathologic scarring after burn wounds. Archives of Facial Plastic Surgery. 2008;**10**:93-102

[35] Singer AJ, Clark RA. Cutaneous wound healing. The New England Journal of Medicine. 1999;**341**:738-746

[36] Arima J, Huang C, Rosner B, Akaishi S, Ogawa R. Hypertension: A systemic key to understanding local keloid severity. Wound Repair and Regeneration. 2015;**23**:213-221

[37] Maligieri LAO, Neves LMG, de Morais DT, Domingues RF, de Aro AA, Pimentel ER, do Amaral MEC, Esquisatto MAM, Dos Santos GMT, Mendonça FAS. Differing energy

densities with laser 670 nm InGaP controls inflammation and collagen reorganization in burns. Burns. Aug 1, 2017 pii: S0305-4179(17)30224-3

[38] Ogawa R. Keloid and hypertrophic scars are the result of chronic inflammation in the Reticuler dermis. International Journal of Molecular Sciences. Mar 10 2017;**18**(3)

[39] Deitch EA, Wheelahan TM, Rose MP, Clothier J, Cotter J. Hypertrophic burn scars: Analysis of variables. The Journal of Trauma. 1983;**23**:895-898

[40] Slemp AE, Kirschner RE. Keloids and scars: A review of keloids and scars, their pathogenesis, risk factors, and management. Current Opinion in Pediatrics. 2006;**18**:396-402

[41] Bombaro KM, Engrav LH, Carrougher GJ, Wiechman SA, Faucher L, Costa BA, Heimbach DM, Rivara FP, Honari S. What is the prevalence of hypertrophic scarring following burns? Burns. 2003;**29**:299-302

[42] Niessen FB, Schalkwijk J, Vos H, et al. Hypertrophic scar formation is associated with an increased number of epidermal Langerhans cells. The Journal of Pathology. 2004; **202**(1):121-129

[43] Correria-Sa I, Serrao P, Marques M, Vieira-Coelho MA. Hypertrophic scars: Are vitamins and inflammatory biomarkers related with the pathophysiology of wound healing? Obesity Surgery. 2017 Jun 1

[44] Schneider JC, Holvanahalli R, Helm P, Goldstein R, Kowalske K. Contractures in burn injury:Defining the problem. Journal of Burn Care & Research. 2006;**27**:508-514

[45] Roberts AB, Sporn MB, Assoian RK, Smith JM, Roche NS, Wakefield LM, Heine UI, Liotta LA, Falanga V, Kehrl JH, Fauci AS. Transforming growth factor-β: Rapid induction of fibrosis and angiogenesis in vivo and stimulation of collagen formation in vitro. Proceedings of the National Academy of Sciences of the United States of America. 1986;**83**:4167-4171

[46] Atiyeh BS. Nonsurgical management of hypertrophic scars: Evidence-based therapies, standard practices,and emerging methods. Aesthetic Plastic Surgery. 2007;**31**:468-494

[47] Moyer KE, Saggers GC, Ehrlich HP. Mast cells promote fibroblast populated collagen lattice contraction through gap junction intercellular communication. Wound Repair and Regeneration. 2004;**12**:269-275

[48] Kopp J, Preis E, Said H, Hafemann B, Wickert L, Gressner AM, Pallua N, Dooley S. Abrogation of transforming growth factor-beta signaling by SMAD7 inhibits collagen gel contraction of human dermal fibroblasts. The Journal of Biological Chemistry. Jun 3, 2005;**280**(22):21570-21576

[49] Johnson-Wint B. Do keratinocytes regulate fibroblast collagenase activities during morphogenesis. Annals of the New York Academy of Sciences. 1998;**548**:167-173

[50] Wang R, Ghahary A, Shen Q, Scott PG, Roy K, Tredget EE. Hypertrophic scar tissues and fibroblasts produce more transforming growth factor-beta 1 mRNA and protein than normal skin and cells. Wound Repair and Regeneration. 2000;**8**:128-137

Section 3

Inflammatory Response In Burn Injury

Chapter 3

The Role of the Inflammatory Response in Burn Injury

Xanthe L. Strudwick and Allison J. Cowin

Additional information is available at the end of the chapter

http://dx.doi.org/10.5772/intechopen.71330

Abstract

Burns are characterised by significant local swelling and redness around the site of injury, indicative of acute inflammation. Whilst the inflammatory response is fundamental to the healing process, triggering a cascade of cytokines and growth factors to protect against the risk of infection, it is clear that prolonged inflammation can be detrimental and lead to scarring and fibrosis. Severe burns may display chronic, persistent inflammation long after the initial burn injury and may even result in multiple organ failure (MOF) due to systemic inflammatory response syndrome (SIRS). Excessive inflammation in the early stages of healing has been identified as a causative factor in the formation of scars which can be disfiguring, functionally restrictive and may require revisionary surgeries. Therefore, it is imperative that inflammation is effectively managed following burn injuries in order to optimise the benefits it provides whilst actively preventing the complications of inflammation including SIRS, multiple organ failure (MOF) and the development of scarring and fibrosis. Reviewing the current knowledge about the role of the inflammatory response in burns and the treatments available for the management of inflammation during wound healing, highlights the importance of continued research into understanding and developing new approaches to regulate inflammatory responses post-burn injuries.

Keywords: burns, inflammation, systemic inflammatory response syndrome, scarring, fibrosis

1. Introduction

In assessing the role of inflammation in burn injuries, it is important to first recognise differences in the pathophysiology of burns. Unlike other wounds, burns consist of three zones of injury, initially described by Jackson in the British Journal of Surgery in 1953. These are the zone of coagulation, the zone of stasis and the zone of hyperaemia [1] (**Figure 1**).

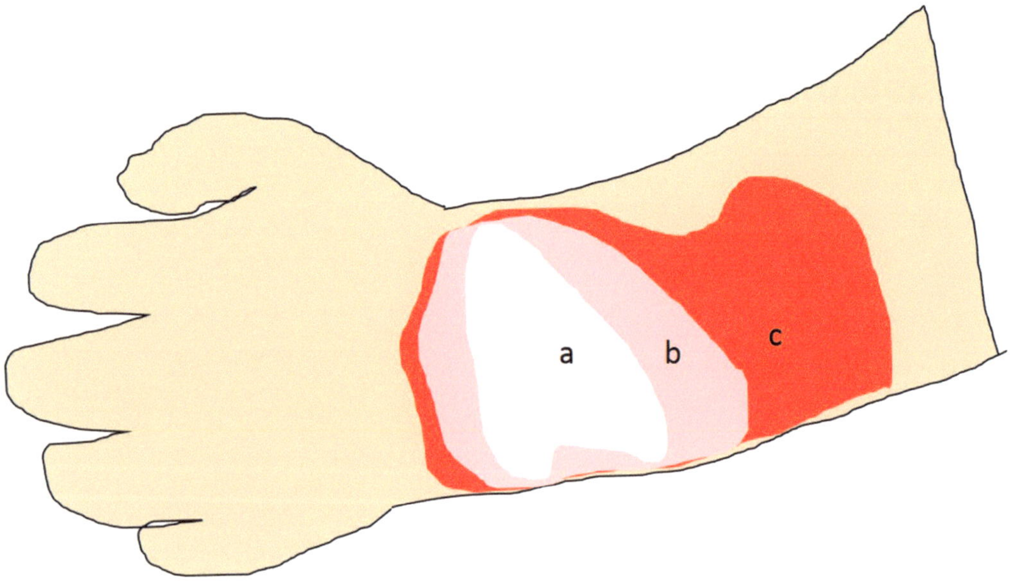

Figure 1. Scald burn in a child showing the Jackson's three zones of damage. (a) Zone of coagulation, (b) zone of stasis and (c) zone of hyperemia. Reproduced from [2].

The primary site of injury, classified as the zone of coagulation, is the site of the most damage and will rapidly undergo necrosis. Outside of this zone, is the zone of stasis that is characterised by reduced blood flow or ischemia and further out, the zone of hyperaemia where microvasculature is not damaged but displays increased blood flow and significant inflammation [2]. If inflammation and vascularisation are not quickly returned to normal, the zone of stasis may also undergo necrosis meaning that the size of the wound may in fact enlarge over time [3]. Thus, the direction of injury in burns is predominantly horizontal as opposed to the vertical injury of an incisional wound [4]. Whilst burn injuries differ from other wound types in that they are sterile at the time of injury, rapid blistering and necrosis of the injured tissue soon opens the wound up to pathogens and the risk of infection [2]. Burns wounds are often larger than other types of wounds, particularly those arising from scalds or exposure to flame and burn injuries covering greater than 20% of the total body area can quickly lead to burn shock due to widespread oedema and fluid loss [5]. The immune status of the patient is also altered following severe burn injuries further contributing to the risk of infection [6]. Thus, infections can quickly overcome a patient if not effectively controlled. It may be for this reason that the inflammatory response in burns is so intense. Moreover, the activity of the immune cells is often dictated by the specific signals encountered within the microenvironment at the site of inflammation or injury [7]. So understanding the factors which alter the protein pathways which are altered in burn wounds is pivotal in the development of therapies to restore balance to the immune response in burn patients and support effective healing of the wound.

2. Inflammation and the healing cascade

Burn injuries initially present with local swelling (oedema) and redness (erythema) around the site of injury (**Figure 1**). More severe, second or third degree burns, which affect more than the superficial epidermis, are characterised by greater levels of oedema and erythema, alongside the formation of blisters and inflammation [2]. This inflammation is indicative of the active immune response which is an integral part of the wound healing cascade, however, it can be significantly elevated in severe burn patients [5, 8]. Although the source of the injury may differ, the phases of wound healing are generally similar and can be described as phases of haemostasis and inflammation, proliferation and remodelling [9] (**Figure 2**). These interrelated and overlapping phases normally progress over a matter of days or weeks to effectively heal a wound, although the timings are often different between types of wounds [10]. In acute wounds, the inflammatory phase lasts for the first 5–7 days, however, severe burns may display chronic, persistent inflammation long after the initial tissue damage and may even result in multiple organ failure (MOF) due to systemic inflammatory response syndrome (SIRS) [11, 12]. Moreover, dysregulation of the inflammatory response and the subsequent progression through the phases of healing are associated with sub-optimal wound outcomes and excessive inflammation can lead to large, thick and restrictive scars [13, 14]. Thus, understanding the interaction between the early inflammatory phase and the later proliferative and remodelling phases of healing are important for understanding the particular complications which may arise following burn injury.

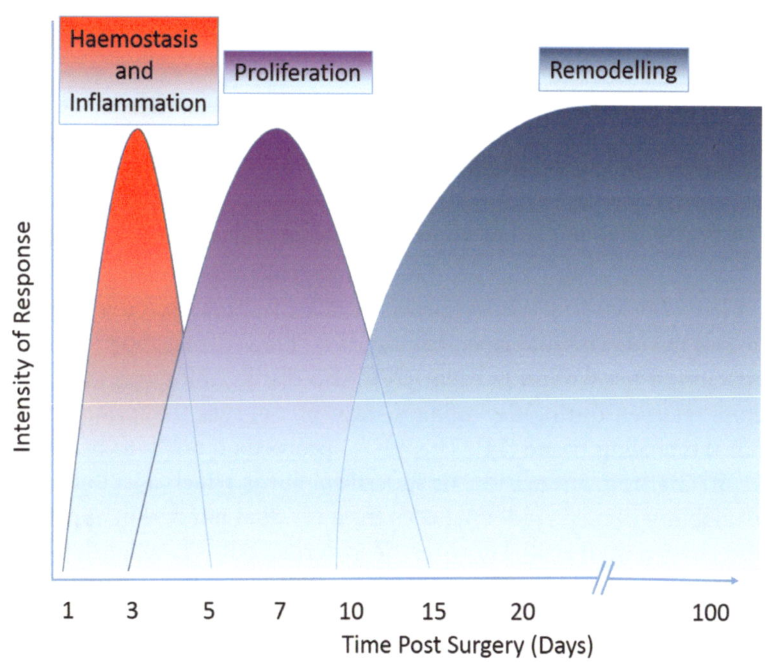

Figure 2. Schematic diagram of the three phases of the healing cascade.

2.1. Haemostasis and inflammation

Immediately following burn injury, haemostasis and coagulation occurs through the formation of a blood clot of platelets and cross-linked fibrin and fibronectin to quickly prevent excessive fluid loss from the wound site [15, 16]. Injured vasculature rapidly constricts to stem blood flow from the open vessels and later vasodilate to facilitate the entrance of blood cells to the wound site needed in the inflammatory phase [9]. Whilst burn wounds exhibit less blood loss than incisional wounds due to heat-induced tissue coagulation, there is still significant damage to the vasculature, with vasoconstriction extending out from the initial injury zone and into the zone of stasis [17]. Moreover, these early stages following burn injury may be complicated by continued damage due to the process of necrosis leading to a significant delay in healing [3, 4]. In all wounds though, key immune cells are recruited to the wound site by signals released from degranulating platelets within the injured tissue [18]. Within hours, the early inflammatory stage begins with the influx of immune cells to the wound site. These cells are responsible for protection from infections, clearance of necrotic and damaged tissue from the wound site and the stimulation of the cells required for repair of the wound during the proliferative and remodelling phases of wound healing [19]. Activated platelets aggregating at the ends of damaged vessels also release growth factors, such as platelet-derived growth factor (PDGF) and transforming growth factor-beta 1 (TGF-β1), to initiate fibroblasts and mesenchymal cells migration from surrounding the wound tissue which will be required for the formation of new extracellular matrix and dermal tissue during the proliferative phase of wound healing [9, 11].

2.2. Proliferation

During the proliferative phase of healing, cells of the epidermis and dermis, the keratinocytes and fibroblasts, proliferate and migrate into the wound site to form the neo-epidermis, restoring barrier function and produce new extracellular matrix which will reconstitute the damaged dermis following injury [19, 20]. The fibroblasts migrate along the fibrin-fibronectin plug into the wound site where they synthesise collagen and elastin and begin remaking the extracellular matrix (ECM) [19]. Whilst fibroblasts migrate into the wound site and form granulation tissue and the new dermal layer, keratinocytes crawl across the provisional matrix for re-epithelialization of the wound to occur [20]. Also during this time, angiogenesis, stimulated by factors released during the inflammatory phase, sees the formation of new blood vessels within the healing tissue [14]. This phase proceeds quickly to heal vertical injuries such as those arising from an incision, or superficial burns which affect only the epidermis, due to the availability of new epidermal cells from residual intact skin appendages residing within the undamaged dermis [4]. However, deep dermal burns heal much slower because of the loss of these skin appendages and reepithelialisation, which can only occur from the edges of the wound, does not begin until the progression of necrosis is halted [21]. Endothelial cells which form new capillary sprouts also interact with the ECM within the wound site, initially producing a dense microvascular network and later, as the levels of collagen increase, reduce the number of blood vessels leaving the resultant tissue with vascularisation levels similar to that of the original tissue [22, 23].

2.3. Remodelling

During the final, remodelling phase of healing, newly formed ECM deposited by fibroblasts is reformed and contracted by myofibroblasts, a process which continues long after the wound appears to be healed and the process of re-epithelialisation is complete [24]. Growth factors released during the inflammatory phase are key to the differentiation of fibroblasts into myofibroblasts [25] and it is the exertion of force by these differentiated, α-smooth muscle actin (α-SMA) positive fibroblasts, upon collagen fibres in the ECM which narrows the margins of the wound assisting wound closure [23, 24]. It is during this final phase of wound healing that the scar tissue is formed. Again, in burn wounds, the remodelling phase is significantly extended, often leading to the formation of hypertrophic scarring and contracture [2]. Initially, fibroblasts deposit type III collagen in the wound, however, as the tissue matures this is replaced by collagen I and collagen fibres are cross-linked to increase the tensile strength of the tissue [26]. A family of matrix metalloproteinases (MMPs), degrade collagen and other ECM components and have key roles in many of the phases of wound healing [27]. Once an equilibrium between collagen deposition and degradation is reached, the scar is considered mature although the organisation of the collagen fibres may continue to be remodelled for many years [13]. Along with this ECM remodelling, apoptosis of immune cells, endothelial cells, keratinocytes, fibroblasts and myofibroblasts and their subsequent clearance from the wound determines the final appearance of the healed tissue [28, 29]. Under normal healing conditions, myofibroblasts will undergo apoptosis and leave the wound site once re-epithelialisation has completed. However, in burn wounds this fails to occur with increased numbers of myofibroblasts observed within the dermis of the scar and fibrosis or pathological contracture ensues [29, 30]. Excessive matrix deposition combined with reduced remodelling are the hallmarks of fibrotic healing, such as is observed in hypertrophic scarring which often occurs following severe burns [26].

In addition to the important role of the inflammatory response in triggering the proliferative and remodelling phases, dysregulation of the inflammatory phase can result in excessive scar formation [10]. The inflammatory response therefore, is clearly fundamental to successful healing of the burn injury. Understanding the immune response, the roles of the specific immune cells and the cytokines and chemokines expressed by these cells within the healing wound is therefore key to understanding how to treat burn injuries and avoid complications due to dysregulation in the inflammatory response.

3. Key immune cells and protein expression in the healing burn wound

Key immune cells are required to present quickly to the burn injury. Whilst some are dermal resident cells, the majority are recruited from the circulation and crawl out of the vasculature into the site of injury [25]. The main inflammatory cells responsible for promoting burn injury repair are mast cells, neutrophils, monocytes and macrophages, whose activities are mediated by a number of the growth factors and signalling proteins (or cytokines) responsible for directing the progression through the healing cascade that are secreted by the immune cells themselves [10]. These ensure both the correct localisation of the required cells within the injured tissue and stimulate the cells to proliferate or differentiate as required to heal the burn. Initially, chemokines, a subset of cytokines, which induce chemotaxis, are expressed following strict spatial and temporal patterns to ensure correct phase-specific recruitment and trafficking of immune cells to the wound site [31]. The expression of growth factors and cytokines further stimulate these immune cells, and other wound active cells, such as the fibroblast and keratinocyte, to carry the out the processes required for burn injury repair [11].

3.1. Mast cells

Burn injury stimulates mast cell degranulation [32, 33] and causes almost instantaneous secretion of histamine and cytokines by tissue resident mast cells [34]. Mast cells are tissue resident cells which play a role in both innate and acquired immunity, through the production histamine, to mediate allergic reaction and are responsible for hypersensitivity reactions [35]. However, these cells are also the first responders following tissue injury, promoting healing during the inflammatory phase where they release cytokines and chemokines, including not only histamine, but also tumour necrosis factor-α (TNF-α), prostaglandins, interleukin (IL)-1, and IL-6, to increase vascular permeability and recruit neutrophils and monocytes to the wound site when stimulated by heat or mechanical trauma [35, 36]. As well as releasing the pro-inflammatory cytokines, mast cells release proteases, such as chymase, which stimulates fibroblasts to migrate into the wound and is associated with fibrosis via its role in stimulating the expression and conversion of TGF-β1 and MMP-9 to their active forms [37]. Mast cells are also found to produce reactive oxygen species (ROS), which despite being an important stimulant of wound healing, excessive or prolonged production of ROS is detrimental to repair. Indeed, the microvascular injury characteristic of burn injuries is likely caused by ROS [32]. In addition to being an important catalyst for wound repair, mast cells may be further recruited to the wound site later in the healing cascade, migrating in from nearby connective tissue or differentiating from circulating basophils [11, 35] and producing tissue plasminogen activator and its antagonist, plasminogen activator inhibitor-1, as well as vascular endothelial growth factor (VEGF), fibroblast growth factor (FGF) and PDGF to modulate both the clotting response and remodelling of the ECM [37]. Likewise, they can release the anti-inflammatory protein IL-10 which helps to dampen an excessive immune response [38]. Thus, mast cells help to fine tune wound healing, depending on temporal and local concentration of the cytokines released by them within the healing tissue.

3.2. Neutrophils

Burn wounds are characterised by persistently high numbers of neutrophils, however, studies have shown that neutrophil chemotaxis is impaired following burn injury, with a reduced directional migration speed, impaired phagocytic function and reduced bactericidal capacity [39–42]. Neutrophils also help clear devitalised tissue through the production of MMPs, collagenase and elastase, clearing the way for the formation of new ECM [8]. These cells also express pro-inflammatory cytokines TNF-α, IL-1β and IL-6 which provide further signals to more neutrophils and other immune cells, such as the monocytes and macrophages, to collect at the wound site [8].

A number of mechanisms are employed by neutrophils to clear infectious agents which include phagolysosomes, the release of free radicals such as ROS and antimicrobial proteases to damage cell membranes and by trapping microbes within nets of histone and DNA [8, 11].

3.3. Monocytes and macrophages

Monocytes and macrophages are often thought as the most important of the immune cells, with important roles in tissue repair and particular alterations in activity following burn injury [43]. Monocytes are a subset of white blood cells which are rapidly recruited to the site of infection or injury from the circulatory system [44]. Here, they may transiently persist as monocytes secreting pro-inflammatory and angiogenic factors, or differentiate into macrophages to support tissue resident macrophages at the wound site to begin clearing the site of extracellular debris, such as damaged matrix, along with fibrin, spent platelets and neutrophils [7, 11]. Both monocytes and macrophages can have pro- or anti-inflammatory effects, often beginning as pro-inflammatory mediators [8]. Initially, most monocytes and macrophages present within the wound site exert pro-inflammatory effects, with an M1 phenotype, and transition to an anti-inflammatory or M2 phenotype later to resolve inflammation, stimulating angiogenesis and progression through the healing cascade [8, 44]. M1 macrophages are the main source of the pro-inflammatory mediators of prostaglandin E2, reactive oxygen and nitrogen intermediates, TNFα, IL-1, IL-6 and IL-8 within the wound to amplify the immune response [8, 43]. M2 macrophages, however, produce an IL-1 receptor antagonist to regulate this response and further produce PDGF, TGF-β1 and FGF to stimulate ECM production and angiogenesis within the newly formed tissue [8, 31, 43]. In burns, there is are significant differences in macrophage populations, with both an initial increase M1 activity, but also a concomitant increase in M2 signalling later in the inflammatory phase [8, 43].

3.4. DAMPs and PAMPs

Some of the earliest signalling pathways to facilitate the wound repair process are triggered by the presence of damage-associated molecular patterns (DAMPs) within the injured tissue. These DAMPs include small molecules, such as ATP, adenosine and bioactive lipids leaked from damaged cells [11]. Studies have shown that a range of DAMPs are significantly elevated immediately following burn injury, due to the significant necrosis induced by burns, which in turn contributes to the excessive monocyte/macrophage activation characteristic of burns [45]. Where infectious agents are also introduced into the wound, these DAMPs are also accompanied by pathogen-associated molecular patterns (PAMPs) such as peptides cleaved from bacterial proteins [7, 11]. Thus, the inflammatory response stimulated by DAMPs found following sterile tissue damage, such as the initial burn insult, can be further exacerbated by PAMPs in infected wounds [7]. PAMPs stimulate the nuclear factor kappa-B (NF-κB) and interferon (IFN) pathways leading to significant upregulation of the cellular immune response to defend against microbial infection [8]. The DAMPs and PAMPs are quickly joined by histamines released from degranulating mast cells, and the growth factors PDGF and TGF-β1 released from platelets [11]. Ischemic injury, such as is present following burn injury, can stimulate additional effects due to the hypoxic environment and reactive oxygen species [7]. Together, these powerful signals trigger the active immune response and result in a strong presence of neutrophils and M1 macrophages and a heightened cellular immune response within the burn wound. In particular, the expression of TNF-α, IL-1, IL-6 and IL-8 by these cells is fundamental to the amplification of the immune response, via the activation of NF-κB and attraction of increasing numbers of immune cells into the wound site [8].

3.5. Complement activation

Burn injury causes systemic upregulation of complement and C-reactive proteins (CRP), enhancing the risk of SIRS and also negatively affecting the healing of the burn [42]. The complement cascades play a key role in the acute phase of the immune response. Part of the innate immune response, the complement system is made up of a number of complement (C) proteins which enhance the ability to fight infection by both directly and indirectly attacking microbes and clearing debris [46]. The complement system is dynamically involved with the cellular immune response, operating via different pathways including the classical, lectin and alternate pathways or via properdin and thrombin, triggered by antibodies expressed on apoptotic cells or microbes, by distinct carbohydrate and lipid residues on injured cells and by DAMPs and PAMPs in the wound site [37, 47–49]. Whilst the different pathways are employed, all complement cascades act to lyse microbes via the formation of C5b and C9 into the membrane attack complex and converge to produce C3a which together with C5 attracts inflammatory cells and promotes phagocytosis and clearance of damaged cells by macrophages [42, 47]. Degranulation of platelets activates the C5 protein [50]. C5, along with C3, in turn stimulate mast cells and thus the complement cascade can modulate mast cell involvement in the resolution of the blood clot and ECM remodelling [37]. Following burn injury, CRP and C3d levels are increased within the local wound site and this increase persists long after the initial injury. The increase in complement is also associated with increased number of macrophages and neutrophils, indicating that the local immune response in burns persists locally much longer than other types of acute wounds [42]. Indeed, it appears that the entire immune system are dynamically involved in the process of burn wound healing.

4. Duality of the immune response in burns patients

The two phases of the inflammatory response are of particular concern following burn injury due to the profound systemic effects upon the patient. Rather than remaining a local response, the initial enhanced pro-inflammatory phase may lead to multiple organ failure and even death as a result of the systemic inflammatory response. Additionally, this can then be followed by an anti-inflammatory phase which often leads to complications for the immunocompromised patient [12]. The greatest difficulty for the treatment of burns lies in the paradox that an active immune response is required for the progression of wound healing and the control of infection, and yet following the excessive initial pro-inflammatory response, increasing the risk of infection due to immune suppression [12, 51, 52]. Thus, the regulation of the intensity and length of the pro-inflammatory and subsequent anti-inflammatory response is of particular importance in burn wound management.

4.1. Systemic inflammatory response syndrome

Excessive immune activation can lead to a systemic inflammatory response syndrome (SIRS) culminating in distant tissue damage and multiple organ dysfunction with the very great risk of death. When pro-inflammatory cytokines, produced during the local immune response that promote the vascular permeability needed for immune cell infiltration, are released into the circulation, they may attack the integrity of distant blood vessels, allowing blood to flood end organs leading to organ failure [51]. Within hours, the increased capillary permeability can lead to hypovolemic shock due to massive fluid loss and requires immediate fluid resuscitation to prevent death [6]. Moreover, intestinal permeability which occurs following severe burns may itself be the source of the inflammatory signalling that causes distant tissue damage [12, 53]. Excessive neutrophilic inflammation is an early hallmark of SIRS but there is significant involvement of the macrophage during the initial phase of the inflammatory response, particularly mediated by their production of pro-inflammatory cytokines TNFα, and IL-6 [43, 52]. As with other severe injuries such as femoral fraction with blood loss greater than 40%, the macrophages in burns appear hyperactive with increased capacity for the production of pro-inflammatory mediators. Indeed, elevated systemic levels of IL-6, IL-8, reactive nitrogen intermediates and prostaglandins are detected in burns patients, all of which mediate both local and distant tissue damage [43]. IL-6 has been shown to be quickly upregulated in the plasma of burns patients, peaking within 6 hours post burn [54]. The levels of IL-6 have been shown to be proportional to the size of the burn and persistently high levels of IL-6 post burn injury may be indicative of both the severity of the burn and likelihood of mortality [54, 55]. Therefore at this time, reducing the severity of the immune response is of critical importance, which needs to be managed carefully before it switches to a profoundly anti-inflammatory phase which itself can have significant side effects.

4.2. Anti-inflammatory response syndrome

Within just a few days of the severe burn, the immune response may become significantly depressed resulting in an anti-inflammatory response syndrome (AIRS). TGF-β1 expression initially peaks 1 day post burn injury and it is likely to have a pro-inflammatory role stimulating the migration of monocytes, neutrophils and fibroblasts into the wound [43, 56]. However, TGF-β1 is also anti-inflammatory and a second peak in TGF-β1 is again detected 1–3 weeks post burn injury [56]. Elevated levels of serum TGF-β1 correlate with the post-burn immunosuppression which is fundamental to the progression of systemic infection or sepsis [43]. Severe burn injuries also display increased anti-inflammatory cytokine IL-4 and IL-10 expression, which inhibit M1 macrophages but stimulate M2 macrophages [8, 57]. Serum levels of the anti-inflammatory cytokine IL-10 peak in burns within 2.5 days following burn injury where increased IL-10 levels is associated with reduced resistance to infection [56, 58]. Indeed, high levels of serum IL-10 at 3 days post burn may be a useful clinical marker of increased risk of mortality in septic burns [58]. During this time, the focus of clinical management is the clearance of infection and supporting the immune response rather than continuing to dampen the response in the hopes of protecting from further tissue damage. It is clear then that dysregulation of the inflammatory response poses great risk to mortality and morbidity, however, the immune response following burn injury may pose one further threat, even when wounds heal without the complications of chronic inflammation leading to SIRS or AIRS. This is due to the fact that excessive inflammation in the early stages of healing has been identified as a causative factor in the formation of scarring and fibrosis.

5. Chronic inflammation and burn scar formation

Burn injuries are often characterised by debilitating hypertrophic scarring, often requiring revisionary surgery (**Figure 3**). In children, scar formation following burn injury is of particular concerns, as the growing child will be restricted by non-elastic scars, which when occurring over moving joints can become functionally restrictive [59]. This is due to an excessive synthesis and deposition of ECM alongside the reduced degradation and remodelling of tissue, leading to the dense formation of collagen in long bundles rather than the normal basket weave formation [60]. Scars are also characterised by an absence of skin appendages such as hair follicles, sweat glands and nerves, which results in functional deficiency, loss of ability to regulate body temperature and absence of sensation [61]. Due to the potentially large areas which may be affected by severe scarring following burn injury, the ability to reduce scar formation is of critical importance.

The link between the increased inflammatory response and the formation of scars is well established [61, 62]. It is clear that prolonged and/or excessive inflammation in the early stages of burn injury leads to excessive fibrosis and scarring [63]. In particular, the numbers of macrophages found within a wound at specific times of the healing cascade are associated with the level of fibrosis and scar formation observed [10]. Likewise, elevated TGF-β1 signalling is directly associated with increased collagen deposition and fibrosis within the healed wound

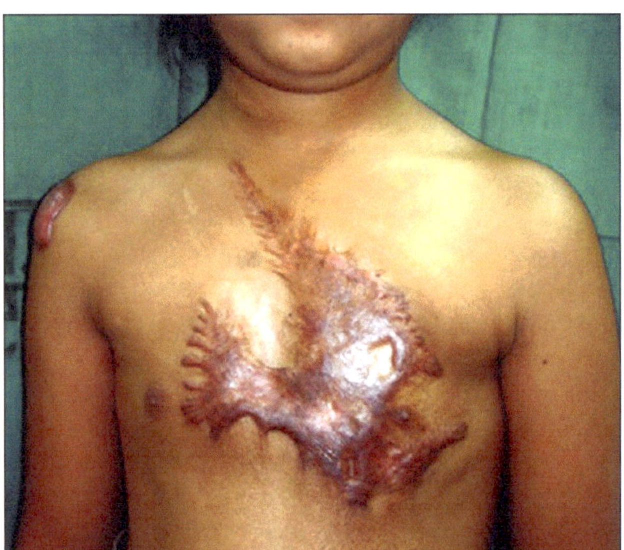

Figure 3. Post-burn hypertrophic scar on anterior chest wall. Reproduced from [59].

as well as myofibroblast over-activation and contracture formation [29, 30, 64]. As described earlier, both the pro-inflammatory macrophage phenotype and elevated TGF-β1 signalling seen in burn wounds contribute to the systemic complication of the immune response as well as this additional role in the formation of hypertrophic scars. There is clearly a very great need for the development of treatments which can control inflammation in burn wounds, to reduce the risk of SIRS and prevent excess scar formation, whilst maintaining the ability to fight infection.

6. Treatments to control inflammation in burns

6.1. Traditional clinical management

Although minor burns heal quickly with little intervention, more severe burns require specialised clinical care to prevent hypovolemic shock, curb inflammation whilst protecting the patient from infection [6, 12]. Fluid resuscitation is often the first step in treating the severe burns patient and research generally centres on determining the optimal fluid volume to avoid cardiac and pulmonary complication, however, the effect of the fluid resuscitation strategy may also impact the inflammatory response [6]. For example, the lactate in a once preferred resuscitation fluid actually stimulates the inflammatory response, negatively affecting the prognosis for burns patients [53]. But the addition of the soluble polysaccharide, glucan phosphate to resuscitation fluid may prove useful as it has been seen to reduce pro-inflammatory cytokine expression post burn whilst increasing resistance to infection by *Pseudomonas aeruginosa* in mice [65]. The nutritional support given to the patient may also modulate the immune system [5]. Indeed, the amounts and specific types of carbohydrates and fats consumed can greatly alter the immune status. It is important to acknowledge then the impact of the dietary changes upon the immune response and investigate how different enteral feeding strategies may impact the immune profile of the patient [5, 66]. For example, a combination of arginine and Omega-3 fatty acid supplementation could be a useful addition due to the initial findings of positive effects on wound healing rates and resistance to infection, but it is not yet known if these will translate into burns patients [67]. A recent clinical trial found that supplementing with isolated soy protein, with or without fish oil was able to decrease the inflammatory response and improve wound healing in burn patients, but it is not yet known which specific compounds in the soy protein are responsible for this action [68]. Interestingly, the topical application of fatty acids isolated from various animals and plants have also been shown to have a positive effect upon burn wound healing and dampening excessive inflammation post burn injury [69], which supports the use of dietary fats in treating burns. However, other adjunct therapies which modulate the immune response have also become the focus of much research into curbing inflammation to reduce mortality and scar formation following burns.

6.2. New research for the modulation of the immune system

A number of avenues for modulating the immune system have so far been investigated which may prove useful in the treatment of burns. These include inhibiting the activation of the immune response, preventing the recruitment and activity of immune cells, interrupting the signalling pathways involved in inflammation and enhancing the resolution of the inflammatory phase.

6.2.1. Inhibition of the activation of the immune response

Curbing inflammation in burns may be achieved at the outset by inhibiting complement activation. Treatment with a C1 inhibitor in a porcine model of burn injury was found to attenuate inflammatory tissue destruction post burn [70, 71] and reduction of C4 in knockout mice prevented hypertrophic scarring following burn injury [72]. Alternatively, blocking immune cell activation using antibodies to block cytokines such as TNFα and IL-1β have been shown to be effective in vitro [52] and local reduction of TNFα using a hyaluronic acid conjugated TNFα antibody reduced necrotic burn progression in a rat model [73]. It has also been suggested that developing therapeutics to prevent NF-κB activation with antioxidants or an agent to block intracellular processes involved in its activation may be a better approach, and there is a current search for a highly specific compound [52]. Stabilisation of mast cells using cromolyn solution prevents both the rise in levels of plasma histamine and xanthine oxidase following thermal injury in rats preventing the initiation of the immune cascade and reducing the severity of the burn [34]. Treatment with pentoxifylline (PTX) immediately following burn injury in mice was found to reduce intestinal permeability and lung injury by reducing levels of intestinal IL-6 and limiting the increase in pro-inflammatory cytokine levels and inflammatory cell activation which may be useful in the prevention of SIRS [53]. Rather than preventing the activation of the immune cells though, one may also aim to reduce their numbers within the wound site.

6.2.2. Prevention of immune cell recruitment and activity

Early studies in mice to deplete numbers of specific immune cells have shown that whilst no one immune cell is critical to wound healing, altering the recruitment or activity of these cells, provided no overt infection pre-exists, may be beneficial to the repair process and indeed may lessen the scarring observed [11]. Studies which specifically depleted macrophage numbers prior to wounding have shown that although wound closure is delayed, the wounds heal with reduced fibrosis and scar formation [74, 75]. Indeed, the targeted depletion of macrophages from the early inflammatory stage (days 0–5) of healing results in minimised scarring. Although these mice showed a reduced rate of epithelialisation during the inflammatory stage, once the mice were allowed to produce new macrophages, wound closure was rapid compared to control animals and with greatly reduced scarring [76]. It has been suggested that reducing the ability of immune cells to receive chemotactic signals may also be useful in modulating the immune response to facilitate better healing [11]. Blocking the activity of chymase released by mast cells using a specific chymase inhibitor TY51469 was effective in supressing neutrophil accumulation, reducing TGF-β1 expression and the extent of pulmonary fibrosis in mice [77] and may be a candidate therapeutic for reducing fibrosis and scarring following severe burns. Indeed, mice which lack mouse mast cell protease (mMCP)-4, the functional equivalent to human chymase, showed a much reduced level of injury following a second-degree scald burn [78].

6.2.3. Interruption of immune signalling pathways

Pharmacological agents which themselves reduce TGF-β1 signalling may also prove useful for reducing fibrosis following burn injury [11]. Alternatively, applying an antibody to interrupt the action of a protein which acts upon the signalling pathway may prove beneficial. The protein Flightless I (Flii) has been shown to modulate TGF-β1 signalling in fibroblasts, with reduced TGF-β1 expression and collagen production in cells with reduced Flii expression [79]. Flii also directly affects the immune response, altering macrophage activation and cytokine production in vitro and increasing Flii expression in diabetic wounds is associated with increased NF-κB production and a prolonged inflammatory phase is observed in the healing of incisional wounds of mice [79–81]. The application of a Flii neutralising antibody in an animal model of the inflammatory skin condition, psoriasis, reduces pro-inflammatory cytokine expression and immune cell infiltration [82]. By treating mouse burn wounds with this antibody and reducing the expression of Flii, it was possible to decrease TGF-β1 levels and cause faster wound healing with less scar formation in mice [83] (**Figure 4**).

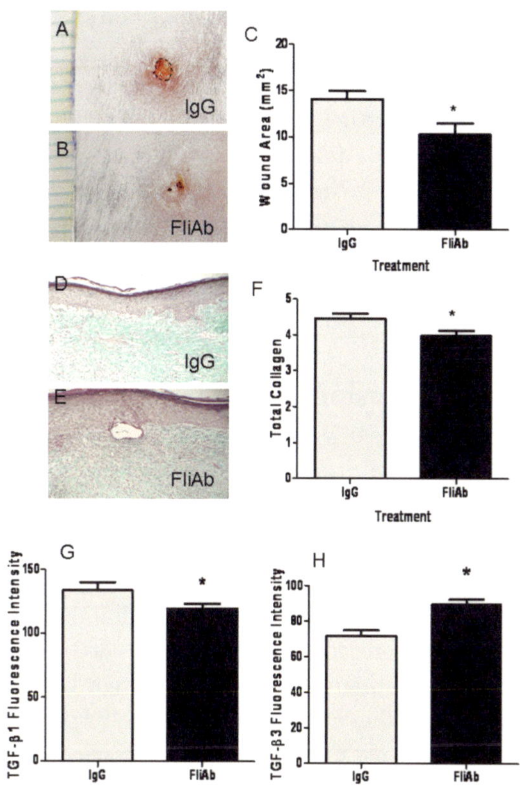

Figure 4. Flii neutralising antibody (FliAb) improves burn injury repair. Representative partial-thickness burn wounds treated with intradermal injection of (a) control IgG (50 μg mL^{-1}) or (b) FliAb (50 μg mL^{-1}) 14 days post-treatment. Dotted line indicates residual burn wound. (c) Graph showing surface wound area of partial-thickness burns treated with either IgG or FliAb post-burn injury. Representative images of (d) IgG and (e) FliAb-treated partial-thickness burns at day 14 post-injury stained with Masson's Trichrome. (f) Graph showing semi-qualitative assessment of total collagen levels within wound of IgG or FliAb-treated burn wounds. (g) Graph showing TGF-β1 fluorescence intensity after 14 days in burn wounds treated with IgG or FliAb post-burn injury. (h) Graph showing TGF-β3 fluorescence intensity after 14 days in burn wounds treated with IgG or FliAb post-burn injury. *Denotes significance $P < 0.05$. Results represent mean ± SEM (n = 8). Reproduced from [83].

The potential therapy has been further investigated in a model of hypertrophic scarring, where it was found that application of Flii antibodies resulted in less fibrosis by reducing the number of myofibroblasts within the wound [84]. Further investigation into the use of neutralising antibodies to dampen inflammation and reduce fibrosis in human burns patients is clearly warranted.

6.2.4. Enhancement of the resolution of the inflammatory response

New therapies are also being developed to resolve post burn inflammation quickly and lead to better healing outcomes. Lipid mediators, such as the resolvins and lipoxins, which stimulate the resolution of the inflammatory phase, have become of particular interest in recent years [11]. Resolvin D2 has recently been found to restore burn neutrophil directionality and can reduce neutrophil numbers and minimise secondary necrosis in burns [85, 86]. The use of phototherapy has been shown to significantly reduce the number of immune cells within a rat burn wound, increasing angiogenesis and collagen deposition [87] and may herald a new area of research for the development of devices to treat burn wounds. Novel biomaterials are also being investigated in the treatment of burn injuries, not only to provide a provisional matrix or augment skin grafting, but are also being assessed for their ability to modulate the immune response [88]. Fibrin-based hydrogels delivered into pig burn wounds prevented contracture but also reduced immune cells within the hydrogel as well as reducing neutrophil and macrophage numbers within the in the surrounding granulation tissue on day 7 post burn [89]. It is expected that future therapies will aim to provide the dual roles of enhancing healing outcomes whilst preventing the excessive systemic inflammatory effects post burn.

7. Considerations and conclusions

Recent studies have revealed some difficulties in predicting and assessing the efficacy of therapies in treating burn wounds. For example, the drugs Atorvastatin and Losartan, originally developed to lower cholesterol levels, showed promise in reducing fibrosis and inflammation in a number of conditions. However, when applied to partial and full thickness burn wounds, it was found that whilst Atrovastatin improved healing of full thickness burns, Losartan was detrimental, but found to be beneficial when applied to partial thickness burns [90]. This highlights the complexities of the immune response and progression through the healing cascade in burn injury and demands that careful consideration be paid during the development of any new therapy to the specific use of a treatment. Moreover, it is not yet known if dampening the immune response by any of these approaches would result in a heightened risk of infection. Therefore investigations into the effect of local versus systemic delivery methods, a thorough understanding of the dose-response effect and confounding effects due to the severity of the injury itself, combined with a careful evaluation of timing of treatments is required. Nevertheless, research into methods, which modulate the immune response, to avoid the complications of a dysregulated immune response and the formation of excess scarring and fibrosis following severe burns remains of critical importance for the future developments of new therapeutic approaches for the treatment of burns.

Author details

Xanthe L. Strudwick and Allison J. Cowin*

*Address all correspondence to: allison.cowin@unisa.edu.au

Regenerative Medicine, Future Industries Institute, University of South Australia, Adelaide, South Australia, Australia

References

[1] Jackson DM. The diagnosis of the depth of burning. The British Journal of Surgery. 1953;**40**(164):588-596

[2] Tiwari VK. Burn wound: How it differs from other wounds? Indian Journal of Plastic Surgery: Official Publication of the Association of Plastic Surgeons of India. 2012;**45**(2): 364-373

[3] Bohr S, Patel SJ, Shen K, Vitalo AG, Brines M, Cerami A, et al. Alternative erythropoietin-mediated signaling prevents secondary microvascular thrombosis and inflammation within cutaneous burns. Proceedings of the National Academy of Sciences. 2013; **110**(9):3513-3518

[4] Linares HA. From wound to scar. Burns. 1996;**22**(5):339-352

[5] Rowan MP, Cancio LC, Elster EA, Burmeister DM, Rose LF, Natesan S, et al. Burn wound healing and treatment: Review and advancements. Critical Care. 2015;**19**:243

[6] Farina JA, Rosique MJ, Rosique RG. Curbing inflammation in burn patients. International Journal of Inflammation. 2013;**2013**:715645

[7] Ogle ME, Segar CE, Sridhar S, Botchwey EA. Monocytes and macrophages in tissue repair: Implications for immunoregenerative biomaterial design. Experimental Biology and Medicine. 2016;**241**(10):1084-1097

[8] Serra MB, Barroso WA, Silva NN, Silva SN, et al. From inflammation to current and alternative therapies involved in wound healing. International Journal of Inflammation. 2017; **2017**:17

[9] Stadelmann WK, Digenis AG, Tobin GR. Physiology and healing dynamics of chronic cutaneous wounds. The American Journal of Surgery. 1998;**176**(2, Supplement 1):26S-38S

[10] Rohl J, Zaharia A, Rudolph M, Murray RZ. The role of inflammation in cutaneous repair. Wound Practice & Research: Journal of the Australian Wound Management Association. 2015;**23**(1):8-12, 4-5

[11] Martin P, Leibovich SJ. Inflammatory cells during wound repair: The good, the bad and the ugly. Trends in Cell Biology. 2005;**15**(11):599-607

[12] Nielson CB, Duethman NC, Howard JM, Moncure M, Wood JG. Burns: Pathophysiology of systemic complications and current management. Journal of Burn Care & Research. 2017; **38**(1):e469-e481

[13] Ehrlich HP, Krummel TM. Regulation of wound healing from a connective tissue perspective. Wound Repair and Regeneration. 1996;**4**(2):203-210

[14] Granger DN, Senchenkova E. Inflammation and the Microcirculation. Integrated Systems Physiology—From Cell to Function. San Rafael (CA): Morgan & Claypool Life Sciences; 2010. Chapter 1, Introduction. Available from: https://www.ncbi.nlm.nih.gov/books/NBK53376/

[15] Clemetson KJ. Platelets and primary haemostasis. Thrombosis Research. 2012;**129**(3):220-224

[16] Wolberg AS, Campbell RA. Thrombin generation, fibrin clot formation and hemostasis. Transfusion and Apheresis Science. 2008;**38**(1):15-23

[17] Shakespeare P. Burn wound healing and skin substitutes. Burns. 2001;**27**(5):517-522

[18] Nguyen D, Orgill D, Murphy G. The pathophysiologic basis for wound healing and cutaneous regeneration. In: Orgill DP, Blanco C, editors. Biomaterials for Treating Skin Loss. Woodhead Publishing Limited; Cambridge: 2009:25-57

[19] Diegelmann RF, Evans MC. Wound healing: An overview of acute, fibrotic and delayed healing. Frontiers in Bioscience. 2004;**9**:283-289

[20] Clark RAF, Lanigan JM, DellaPelle P, Manseau E, Dvorak HF, Colvin RB. Fibronectin and fibrin provide a provisional matrix for epidermal cell migration during wound reepithelialization. Journal of Investigative Dermatology. 1982;**79**(5):264-269

[21] Cuttle L, Kempf M, Phillips GE, Mill J, Hayes MT, Fraser JF, et al. A porcine deep dermal partial thickness burn model with hypertrophic scarring. Burns. 2006;**32**(7):806-820

[22] Tonnesen MG, Feng X, Clark RA. Angiogenesis in wound healing. The Journal of Investigative Dermatology. Symposium Proceedings. 2000;**5**(1):40-46

[23] Amadeu T, Braune A, Mandarim-de-Lacerda C, Porto LC, Desmouliere A, Costa A. Vascularization pattern in hypertrophic scars and keloids: A stereological analysis. Pathology, Research and Practice. 2003;**199**(7):469-473

[24] Amadeu TP, Coulomb B, Desmouliere A, Costa AM. Cutaneous wound healing: Myofibroblastic differentiation and in vitro models. The International Journal of Lower Extremity Wounds. 2003;**2**(2):60-68

[25] Eming SA, Krieg T, Davidson JM. Inflammation in wound repair: Molecular and cellular mechanisms. Journal of Investigative Dermatology. 2007;**127**(3):514-525

[26] Lazarus GS, Cooper DM, Knighton DR, Margolis DJ, Percoraro RE, Rodeheaver G, et al. Definitions and guidelines for assessment of wounds and evaluation of healing. Wound Repair and Regeneration. 1994;**2**(3):165-170

[27] Gill SE, Parks WC. Metalloproteinases and their inhibitors: Regulators of wound healing. International Journal of Biochemistry & Cell Biology. 2008;**40**(6-7):1334-1347

[28] Greenhalgh DG. The role of apoptosis in wound healing. The International Journal of Biochemistry & Cell Biology. 1998;**30**(9):1019-1030

[29] Gabbiani G. The myofibroblast in wound healing and fibrocontractive diseases. The Journal of Pathology. 2003;**200**(4):500-503

[30] Shin D, Minn KW. The effect of myofibroblast on contracture of hypertrophic scar. Plastic and Reconstructive Surgery. 2004;**113**(2):633-640

[31] Engelhardt E, Toksoy A, Goebeler M, Debus S, Brocker EB, Gillitzer R. Chemokines IL-8, GROalpha, MCP-1, IP-10, and Mig are sequentially and differentially expressed during phase-specific infiltration of leukocyte subsets in human wound healing. The American Journal of Pathology. 1998;**153**(6):1849-1860

[32] Santos FX, Arroyo C, García I, Blasco R, Obispo JM, Hamann C, et al. Role of mast cells in the pathogenesis of postburn inflammatory response: Reactive oxygen species as mast cell stimulators. Burns. 2000;**26**(2):145-147

[33] Bankova LG, Lezcano C, Pejler G, Stevens RL, Murphy GF, Austen KF, et al. Mouse mast cell proteases 4 and 5 mediate epidermal injury through disruption of tight junctions. Journal of Immunology. 2014;**192**(6):2812-2820

[34] Friedl HP, Till GO, Trentz O, Ward PA. Roles of histamine, complement and xanthine oxidase in thermal injury of skin. The American Journal of Pathology. 1989;**135**(1):203-217

[35] Douaiher J, Succar J, Lancerotto L, Gurish MF, Orgill DP, Hamilton MJ, et al. Development of mast cells and importance of their Tryptase and Chymase serine proteases in inflammation and wound healing. Advances in Immunology. 2014;**122**:211-252

[36] Wilgus TA, Wulff BC. The importance of mast cells in dermal scarring. Advances in Wound Care. 2014;**3**(4):356-365

[37] Oskeritzian CA. Mast cells and wound healing. Advances in Wound Care. 2012;**1**(1):23-28

[38] Galli SJ, Tsai M. Mast cells: Versatile regulators of inflammation, tissue remodeling, host defense and homeostasis. Journal of Dermatological Science. 2008;**49**(1):7-19

[39] Butler KL, Ambravaneswaran V, Agrawal N, Bilodeau M, Toner M, Tompkins RG, et al. Burn injury reduces neutrophil directional migration speed in microfluidic devices. PLoS One. 2010;**5**(7):e11921

[40] Arturson G. Neutrophil granulocyte functions in severely burned patients. Burns, Including Thermal Injury. 1985;**11**(5):309-319

[41] Calum H, Moser C, Jensen PØ, Christophersen L, Maling DS, van Gennip M, et al. Thermal injury induces impaired function in polymorphonuclear neutrophil granulocytes and reduced control of burn wound infection. Clinical and Experimental Immunology. 2009;**156**(1):102-110

[42] van de Goot F, Krijnen PAJ, Begieneman MPV, Ulrich MMW, Middelkoop E, Niessen HWM. Acute inflammation is persistent locally in burn wounds: A pivotal role for complement and C-reactive protein. Journal of Burn Care & Research. 2009;**30**(2):274-280

[43] Schwacha MG. Macrophages and post-burn immune dysfunction. Burns. 2003;**29**(1):1-14

[44] Olingy CE, San Emeterio CL, Ogle ME, Krieger JR, Bruce AC, Pfau DD, et al. Non-classical monocytes are biased progenitors of wound healing macrophages during soft tissue injury. Scientific Reports. 2017;**7**(1):447

[45] Rani M, Nicholson SE, Zhang Q, Schwacha MG. Damage-associated molecular patterns (DAMPs) released after burn are associated with inflammation and monocyte activation. Burns. 2017;**43**(2):297-303

[46] Janeway CA Jr, Medzhitov R. Innate immune recognition. Annual Review of Immunology. 2002;**20**:197-216

[47] Cazander G, Jukema GN, Nibbering PH. Complement activation and inhibition in wound healing. Clinical & Developmental Immunology. 2012;**2012**:534291

[48] Korkmaz HI, Krijnen PAJ, Ulrich MMW, de Jong E, van Zuijlen PPM, Niessen HWM. The role of complement in the acute phase response after burns. Burns. 2017;**43**(7):1390-1399

[49] Ricklin D, Hajishengallis G, Yang K, Lambris JD. Complement—A key system for immune surveillance and homeostasis. Nature Immunology. 2010;**11**(9):785-797

[50] Sinno H, Malholtra M, Lutfy J, Jardin B, Winocour S, Brimo F, et al. Topical application of complement C3 in collagen formulation increases early wound healing. The Journal of Dermatological Treatment. 2013;**24**(2):141-147

[51] Bone RC. Toward a theory regarding the pathogenesis of the systemic inflammatory response syndrome: What we do and do not know about cytokine regulation. Critical Care Medicine. 1996;**24**(1):163-172

[52] Christman JW, Lancaster LH, Blackwell TS. Nuclear factor kappa B: A pivotal role in the systemic inflammatory response syndrome and new target for therapy. Intensive Care Medicine. 1998;**24**(11):1131-1138

[53] Costantini TW, Peterson CY, Kroll L, Loomis WH, Putnam JG, Wolf P, et al. Burns, inflammation, and intestinal injury: Protective effects of an anti-inflammatory resuscitation strategy. The Journal of Trauma. 2009;**67**(6):1162-1168

[54] Ueyama M, Maruyama I, Osame M, Sawada Y. Marked increase in plasma interleukin-6 in burn patients. The Journal of Laboratory and Clinical Medicine. 1992;**120**(5):693-698

[55] Yeh FL, Lin WL, Shen HD. Changes in circulating levels of an anti-inflammatory cytokine interleukin 10 in burned patients. Burns. 2000;**26**(5):454-459

[56] Yeh FL, Shen HD, Fang RH. Deficient transforming growth factor β and interleukin-10 responses contribute to the septic death of burned patients. Burns. 2002;**28**(7):631-637

[57] O'Sullivan ST, Lederer JA, Horgan AF, Chin DH, Mannick JA, Rodrick ML. Major injury leads to predominance of the T helper-2 lymphocyte phenotype and diminished interleukin-12 production associated with decreased resistance to infection. Annals of Surgery. 1995;**222**(4):482-490 discussion 90-2

[58] Pileri D, Accardo Palombo A, D'Amelio L, D'Arpa N, Amato G, Masellis A, et al. Concentrations of cytokines Il-6 and Il-10 in plasma of burn patients: Their relationship to sepsis and outcome. Annals of Burns and Fire Disasters. 2008;**21**(4):182-185

[59] Goel A, Shrivastava P. Post-burn scars and scar contractures. Indian Journal of Plastic Surgery: Official Publication of the Association of Plastic Surgeons of India. 2010; **43**(Suppl):S63-S71

[60] Dallon J, Sherratt J, Maini P, Ferguson M. Biological implications of a discrete mathematical model for collagen deposition and alignment in dermal wound repair. IMA Journal of Mathematics Applied in Medicine and Biology. 2000;**17**(4):379-393

[61] Aarabi S, Longaker MT, Gurtner GC. Hypertrophic scar formation following burns and trauma: New approaches to treatment. PLoS Medicine. 2007;**4**(9):e234

[62] Singer AJ, Clark RA. Cutaneous wound healing. The New England Journal of Medicine. 1999;**341**(10):738-746

[63] Lucas T, Waisman A, Ranjan R, Roes J, Krieg T, Muller W, et al. Differential roles of macrophages in diverse phases of skin repair. Journal of Immunology. 2010;**184**(7):3964-3977

[64] Martin P. Wound healing—Aiming for perfect skin regeneration. Science. 1997;**276**(5309): 75-81

[65] Lyuksutova OI, Murphey ED, Toliver-Kinsky TE, Lin CY, Cui W, Williams DL, et al. Glucan phosphate treatment attenuates burn-induced inflammation and improves resistance to *Pseudomonas aeruginosa* burn wound infection. Shock. 2005;**23**(3):224-232

[66] Fritsche KL. The science of fatty acids and inflammation. Advances in Nutrition. 2015;**6**(3): 293S-301S

[67] Alexander JW, Supp DM. Role of arginine and Omega-3 fatty acids in wound healing and infection. Advances in Wound Care. 2014;**3**(11):682-690

[68] Babajafari S, Akhlaghi M, Mazloomi SM, Ayaz M, Noorafshan A, Jafari P, et al. The effect of isolated soy protein adjunctive with flaxseed oil on markers of inflammation, oxidative stress, acute phase proteins, and wound healing of burn patients; a randomized clinical trial. Burns. 2017. DOI:10.1016/j.burns.2017.05.014. [Epub ahead of print]

[69] Li X-Q, Kang R, Huo J-C, Xie Y-H, Wang S-W, Cao W. Wound-healing activity of *Zanthoxylum bungeanum* maxim seed oil on experimentally burned rats. Pharmacognosy Magazine. 2017;**13**(51):363-371

[70] Henze U, Lennartz A, Hafemann B, Goldmann C, Kirkpatrick CJ, Klosterhalfen B. The influence of the C1-inhibitor BERINERT and the protein-free haemodialysate

ACTIHAEMYL20% on the evolution of the depth of scald burns in a porcine model. Burns. 1997;**23**(6):473-477

[71] Radke A, Mottaghy K, Goldmann C, Khorram-Sefat R, Kovacs B, Janssen A, et al. C1 inhibitor prevents capillary leakage after thermal trauma. Critical Care Medicine. 2000;**28**(9):3224-3232

[72] Suber F, Carroll MC, Moore FD Jr. Innate response to self-antigen significantly exacerbates burn wound depth. Proceedings of the National Academy of Sciences of the United States of America. 2007;**104**(10):3973-3977

[73] Sun LT, Friedrich E, Heuslein JL, Pferdehirt RE, Dangelo NM, Natesan S, et al. Reduction of burn progression with topical delivery of (anti-tumor necrosis factor-α)-hyaluronic acid conjugates. Wound Repair and Regeneration. 2012;**20**(4):563-572

[74] Mirza R, DiPietro LA, Koh TJ. Selective and specific macrophage ablation is detrimental to wound healing in mice. The American Journal of Pathology. 2009;**175**(6):2454-2462

[75] Goren I, Allmann N, Yogev N, Schurmann C, Linke A, Holdener M, et al. A transgenic mouse model of inducible macrophage depletion: effects of diphtheria toxin-driven lysozyme M-specific cell lineage ablation on wound inflammatory, angiogenic, and contractive processes. American Journal of Pathology. 2009;**175**(1):132-147

[76] Ley K, Laudanna C, Cybulsky MI, Nourshargh S. Getting to the site of inflammation: The leukocyte adhesion cascade updated. Nature Reviews. Immunology. 2007;**7**(9):678-689

[77] Takato H, Yasui M, Ichikawa Y, Waseda Y, Inuzuka K, Nishizawa Y, et al. The specific chymase inhibitor TY-51469 suppresses the accumulation of neutrophils in the lung and reduces silica-induced pulmonary fibrosis in mice. Experimental Lung Research. 2011;**37**(2): 101-108

[78] Younan G, Suber F, Xing W, Shi T, Kunori Y, Abrink M, et al. The inflammatory response following an epidermal burn depends on the activities of mouse mast cell proteases 4 and 5. Journal of immunology (Baltimore, MD: 1950). 2010;**185**(12):7681-7690

[79] Adams DH, Strudwick XL, Kopecki Z, Hooper-Jones JA, Matthaei KI, Campbell HD, et al. Gender specific effects on the actin-remodelling protein flightless I and TGF-beta1 contribute to impaired wound healing in aged skin. The International Journal of Biochemistry & Cell Biology. 2008;**40**(8):1555-1569

[80] Ruzehaji N, Mills SJ, Melville E, Arkell R, Fitridge R, Cowin AJ. The influence of flightless I on toll-like-receptor-mediated inflammation in a murine model of diabetic wound healing. BioMed Research International. 2013;**2013**:389792

[81] Lei N, Franken L, Ruzehaji N, Offenhauser C, Cowin AJ, Murray RZ. Flightless, secreted through a late endosome/lysosome pathway, binds LPS and dampens cytokine secretion. Journal of Cell Science. 2012;**125**(Pt 18):4288-4296

[82] Chong HT, Yang GN, Sidhu S, Ibbetson J, Kopecki Z, Cowin AJ. Reducing flightless I expression decreases severity of psoriasis in an imiquimod-induced murine model of psoriasiform dermatitis. The British Journal of Dermatology. 2017;**176**(3):705-712

[83] Adams DH, Ruzehaji N, Strudwick XL, Greenwood JE, Campbell HD, Arkell R, et al. Attenuation of flightless I, an actin-remodelling protein, improves burn injury repair via modulation of transforming growth factor (TGF)-beta1 and TGF-beta3. The British Journal of Dermatology. 2009;**161**(2):326-336

[84] Cameron AM, Turner CT, Adams DH, Jackson JE, Melville E, Arkell RM, et al. Flightless I is a key regulator of the Fibroproliferative process in hypertrophic scarring and a target for a novel anti-scarring therapy. The British Journal of Dermatology. 2015

[85] Kurihara T, Jones CN, Yu Y-M, Fischman AJ, Watada S, Tompkins RG, et al. Resolvin D2 restores neutrophil directionality and improves survival after burns. The FASEB Journal. 2013;**27**(6):2270-2281

[86] Inoue Y, Liu YM, Otawara M, Chico Calero I, Stephanie Nam A, Yu Y-M, et al. Resolvin D2 limits secondary tissue necrosis after burn wounds in rats. Journal of burn care & research: official publication of the American Burn Association. 2017

[87] Maligieri LAO, Neves LMG, de Morais DT, Domingues RF, de Aro AA, Pimentel ER, et al. Differing energy densities with laser 670nm InGaP controls inflammation and collagen reorganization in burns. Burns. 2017. DOI: 10.1016/j.burns.2017.04.008. Epub 2017 Aug 1

[88] Rahimnejad M, Derakhshanfar S, Zhong W. Biomaterials and tissue engineering for scar management in wound care. Burns & Trauma. 2017;**5**(1):4

[89] Burmeister DM, Roy DC, Becerra SC, Natesan S, Christy RJ. Situ delivery of fibrin-based hydrogels prevents contraction and reduces inflammation. Journal of Burn Care & Research: Official Publication of the American Burn Association. 2017

[90] Akershoek JJ, Brouwer KM, Vlig M, Boekema BKHL, Beelen RHJ, Middelkoop E, et al. Differential effects of losartan and atorvastatin in partial and full thickness burn wounds. PLoS One. 2017;**12**(6):e0179350

Section 4

Treatment of Burn Injury

Chapter 4

The Therapeutic Effects of Conservative Treatments on Burn Scars

Mehmet Unal

Additional information is available at the end of the chapter

http://dx.doi.org/10.5772/intechopen.70833

Abstract

Hypertrophic scar, which can be seen even after minor burn injuries, is a common complication and generally develops within 6–8 weeks following reepithelization. Hypertrophic scar/keloid is often seen when the injury affects the reticular dermis and, in particular, after a deep dermal or full thickness burn. There are various options used in the treatment of burn scar. The purpose of this chapter is to provide the reader a brief information on the conservative treatment methods used in burn scar treatment.

Keywords: burn injury, hypertrophic scar, keloid, burn scar, conservative treatment

1. Introduction

Animals developed a generally well-functioning pathway in the healing of damaged tissues. While some species have the ability to regenerate damaged or missing tissues, it is rare for people. Only the epidermis has full regeneration capacity, after the second trimester of fetal development, so any damage involving the dermis always heals with a scar. In humans, wounds usually heal with a normal scar, and hypertrophic scar process is not common. In some cases, the scar overcomes the original injury and results in the lesion known as keloid. Both hypertrophic scars and keloids cause a significant discomfort and malformation.

Although we believe that the word of "keloid" was first used by Aliberti in the nineteenth century, there were hypertrophic scar and keloid definitions among ancient Egypt hieroglyphs [1].

1.1. Epidemiology

Keloid and hypertrophic scars can occur all over the world and in all skin types. The risk of keloid formation increases as the skin color becomes darker, and the incidence of keloid in the Black population was found as high as 16%. Keloid develops equally in both men and women. Although reported in all ages, it is rare in young children and elderly people. It is thought that there is a familial predisposition for hypertrophic scarring and keloid development. Although previous reports have implied an autosomal recessive inheritance pattern, an autosomal dominant transition with incomplete clinical penetrance and variable expression was considered in a recent review. Two rare syndromes involving spontaneous keloid development are Rubinstein-Taybi and Goeminne syndromes [2, 3].

1.2. Pathogenesis

The pathogenesis of hypertrophic scarring and keloid formation is unknown. In patients with hypertrophic scars and keloids, wound healing process shifts in a different direction than normal, and spontaneous involution does not generally occur. Its cause is unknown, but events such as infections, extreme wound tightness, and foreign bodies that are known to trigger for inflammation have been emphasized in the keloid development.

Melanocytes may play a role in the development of hypertrophic scar, because keloids have not been reported in patients with oculocutaneous albinism and keloids are more common in dark-skinned individuals. Mast cells are found intensely in hypertrophic scars and keloids. Mast cell mediators regulate collagen synthesis and are known to contribute to excessive accumulation.

Transforming growth factor-B (TGF-B) appears to be another molecule that causes scarring and keloid formation, because both transforming growth factor-B (TGF-B)-1 and TGF-B-2 are produced more from fibroblasts in keloid tissue than in normal fibroblasts [1–5].

1.3. Clinical features

Hypertrophic scars and keloids have many common features. Both are rough, often painful, itchy, pink-purple lesions. The epidermis is typically flat and the dermal part of the lesion is felt hard with palpation. Hypertrophic scars and keloids are malformed and may prevent normal movement of the surrounding tissues. Hypertrophic scars and keloids may appear anywhere of body, but especially ear lobe, upper part of body, and deltoid region are more risky areas. On the other hand, keloids are rare in the middle of the face, eyelids, and genital area.

Although hypertrophic scars and keloids usually appear after a trauma, they can also develop spontaneously. Before the onset of hypertrophic scars and keloids, various skin injuries such as acne, infection, burns, and piercing can be found. Clinical findings of lesions distinguish hypertrophic scars from keloids. Although hypertrophic scars remain in the area of original damage and tend to regress progressively over time, keloids tend to slowly heal in the middle parts, but tend to invade the surrounding tissues [1, 2].

1.4. Pathology

Both hypertrophic scars and keloids have increased cellularity, vascularity, and connective tissue compared to normal skin and normal scar. Hypertrophic scars include myofibroblasts, small vessel walls, and nodules with fine collagen fibrils. Over time, these nodules become thinner and the collagen bands become parallel to the skin surface. Keloids are histologically characterized by large, thick collagen fibers composed of numerous, firmly attached fibrils. An ultrastructurally amorphous extracellular material surrounds the fibroblastic cells in the keloid [5].

1.5. Hypertrophic scar-keloid and burn injury

Hypertrophic scarring/keloid is often seen when the injury affects the reticular dermis and, in particular, after a deep dermal or full thickness burn.

Severe burns caused high mortality rates in the past. The development of specialized burn centers and advances in treatment options have led to more survivors of the burn victim. Due to long hospitalization periods and deprivation of daily physical activity, burn patients suffer from problems such as reduction in muscle strength, limitation of joint movements, and decrease in fitness level. Moreover, hypertrophic scarring, which can be seen even after minor burn injuries, is a common complication and generally develops within 6–8 weeks following reepithelialization. Although children are particularly susceptible to hypertrophic scarring due to the rapid nature of their cell formation, burn scars are common both in children and adults and can result in extensive skin damage [6–8].

There are many different options used in the treatment of burn scar. The purpose of this chapter is to provide the reader a brief information on the conservative treatment methods used in burn scar treatment.

2. Conservative treatments

- Pressure therapy
- Silicone gel therapy
- Hydration
- Ultrasound
- Electroacupuncture
- Onion extract
- Massage therapy
- Combined therapy

2.1. Pressure therapy

Formation of hypertrophic scar (HS) is a common undesirable consequence of trauma directing to the skin [6]. A classical scar is in red-pink or purple color, rigid, and raised and usually together with pain and/or itchiness. Hypertrophic scar that significantly disrupts normal skin functions may lead to further restriction of daily activities [6, 7] and psychosocial troubles among the patients [8–14].

Pressure therapy is considered as the first-line treatment option in improving the appearance of hypertrophic scar and reducing the rate of maturation. The general application way of pressure therapy is pressure garments [11–13]. Pressure therapy, dating back to Ambroise Pare in the sixteenth century, is a treatment that has been used for a long time by different methods. But, the popularity of pressure therapy for hypertrophic burn scars has been increased after successful results with this therapy reported from the Shriners Galveston Burn Hospital. In 1971, burn hospital team from Galveston declared a decrease in hypertrophic scar formation rate after thermal injury with pressure therapy application [13–17].

So far, the mechanism of action of pressure therapy has remained theoretical, and the efficacy and benefits of pressure garments are still a mystery. The optimal pressure level is also still a controversial topic. Theoretically, the minimum pressure to be applied during pressure therapy should be greater than the capillary pressure, meaning that the pressure should be at least 24 mmHg or more. But, there are studies in which 5–15 mmHg pressure was applied and successful clinical results such as less itching, better appearance of the scar, and so on were observed [18]. On the other hand, it was reported that paresthesia and maceration may occur shortly after application of high levels of pressure (over 40 mmHg) [19].

It was showed in studies that application of pressure significantly decreases the thickness of hypertrophic scar and the number of surgical procedures needed for correction. It is still unclear how the pressure has reduced the scar thickness. It is claimed that the pressure provides the rearrangement of collagen fibers, decreases the development of whorled typed collagen nodules, and thus, provokes the softening of scar tissue and the reduction of its thickness [6, 11, 13]. Despite the general acceptance that pressure therapy is effective, there is no clear consensus about the minimum effective amount of pressure. Although partially good results with low pressure values (5–15 mmHg) were reported in previous studies, it is thought that the higher amount of pressure provides more reduction in scar thickness [6, 11, 19]. In their study, Candy et al. observed that high pressure (>20 to 25 mmHg) garment demonstrated its superior effects on reducing scar thickness after 5 months treatment, leading to an overall reduction of 40.05% in thickness and the most prominent improvement was observed after the first month of intervention. Although scars with low pressure treatment also showed significant improvement, for this group overall thickness reduction was 19.79% [6].

The presence of erythema has always been considered as a major marker of hypertrophic scarring after burns. It has been shown that redness is increased in scar tissues which have higher vascularity, determined using Laser Doppler from previous studies [6, 20, 21]. Parallel to this, a reduction in redness/erythema may imply a decrease of vascular flow to the scar tissues [21, 22]; meaning that, the nutrient and oxygen supply for cellular activities was reduced. Hypoxic milieu due to pressure therapy may trigger fibroblasts apoptosis process [20–23]. Although it was reported that higher pressure (>20 to 25 mmHg) values lead to reductions in erythema, the pressure must be at least 24 mmHg or higher to provide a significant reduction [6, 11].

Pressure therapy also improves the hardness of hypertrophic scar and increases pliability, but data on this topic are quite limited [13, 24]. And finally, pressure therapy (only high pressure) causes a significant improvement in pigmentation of scar tissue [6].

The most important problems with the use of pressure therapy are the long duration of treatment and need to wear pressure garment during 14–23 h/day, which reduce the patient's compliance with treatment [24].

An important point to be aware of during pressure therapy is that pressure loss of the garments over time. Pressure garments lose their elasticity over the wearing period. The reason is probably that pressure garments are usually made of spandex and nylon fabric and these materials decrease their elasticity upon prolonged wear. Pressure loss of the garments can lead to treatment failure, so the physician should be careful in this regard [6, 25].

2.2. Silicone gel

Hypertrophic scar emerges as a consequence of an excessive response of the skin to trauma. Hypertrophic scar can cause pain and itching as well as cause cosmetic problems and may restrict range of motion [26].

There is very limited evidence to show the effectiveness of treatments to reduce or prevent scar formation. Most of the available information and recommendations are based on experience of practitioners and small scale studies. Also, there are very limited scientific data on the long-term effects of these treatments. Nevertheless, treatments such as the use of intralesional corticosteroid injections, silicone sheets, occlusive dressings, and custom-made pressure garments have a general acceptance [27].

The earliest known silicone gel sheet was developed by Perkins et al. for use at 6–8 weeks after the initial injury, when the scars started to develop. Since its first use in the early 1980s, silicone gels have a wide use in burn scar treatment. Although the mechanism of how to heal burn scars is not yet fully understood, the noninvasive character of silicone gels makes them easily acceptable for patients in treatment and prophylaxis of hypertrophic scars [26–28].

Studies demonstrated the effectiveness of silicone gels in the treatment of scars, but the mechanism of how to heal scars and physiological effects of silicone gel are not yet fully understood. It is believed that silicone gels affect the stratum corneum by decreasing evaporation and providing a better hemostasis in the scar tissue. Stratum corneum on the hypertrophic scar and keloid tissue causes more evaporation of water from the underlying tissue than in normal skin. Silicone gels reduce evaporation and thus provide an optimal hydration in the stratum corneum. The silicone gels may influence the stratum corneum by inhibiting mast cell activity and reducing edema, vasodilatation, and excessive extracellular matrix synthesis, but perhaps the main mechanism of action of gels may depend on their simpler effects such as changes in temperature, oxygen, pressure, hydration, and tension produced by wound coverage. Another hypothesis is that static electricity on silicone gels may cause the re- alignment of collagen deposition [26, 27, 29–31].

In studies, different types of silicone were used, such as silicone sheets (not specified), cica-care silicone gel sheets, silastic gel sheets, Sil-K silicone, and Epiderm silicone sheets or

Dermatix topical silicone gel in diverse patient populations. Therefore, it is not easy to assess which kind of silicone gels is more effective and optimal [24].

In a prospective randomized clinical trial, the authors applied silicone gel sheeting (SGS) 24 hour per day for 6 months. In this study, subjects with 6-month silicone gel intervention showed a reduction of scar thickness measured by tissue ultrasound palpation system. The scar in the group used silicone gel was softer and more pliable as measured by The Vancouver Scar Scale and there was reduction on pain and itchiness from patients. Although the vascularity and pigmentation did not show any statistical significant difference, individuals in the SGS groups stated that the scar became less reddish, paler, and more resembled normal skin. When compared to the control group, patients in the SGS group also had faster rate of recovery from pain and itchiness, but the results at the 6-month assessment were not different between the two groups [32].

The topical silicone gel was applied twice a day and was typically worn 12–24 h a day, excluding bathing time. The duration of application varies between 12 and 28 weeks [24].

Despite the effectiveness of silicon gels, there are some limitations to their use. Patient compliance can be low when silicone gels are used on scars on visible regions, the appearance can make them less popular for the patient to use, and scar located near to joints, due to their potential restriction of movements and because gels sometimes do not stay adherent on these regions.

In addition, hygiene of gels and involved skin must be considered, especially in hot climates, to avoid irritation or rash and infections [26, 27, 32–34].

2.3. Hydration

When the wound healing reaches enough strength to tolerate skin massage, it is a routine practice to perform a scar massage with a solution that usually contains a moisturizing product [33]. Because hydrating effect of silicone gels on the stratum corneum has been suggested as a mechanism underlying its therapeutic effectiveness, many authors have reported the efficacy of treatment with topical silicone gel sheet for keloids and hypertrophic scars. Additionally, it is recommended that hydration/moisturizing of scar tissue, since transepidermal water loss rates are higher when compared to healthy skin [24, 32, 33].

Various products, including aqueous cream BP, bees wax and herbal oil creams, silicone-based creams, and paraffin/petroleum-based products, have been reported for use in practice as well as in literature on scar management [35].

Aqueous cream BP, which is fragrance and color free, is a readily available and relatively not expensive emollient production. Purified water, white soft paraffin, cetearyl alcohol and sodium lauryl sulfate (SLS), liquid paraffin, and phenoxyethanol are carried in this formulation [35].

Bees wax and herbal oil cream are the other two agents providing a greater decrease in the symptom of itch following burn injury when compared to aqueous cream BP, especially along with the use of antipruritic medications [35, 36].

http://dx.doi.org/10.5772/intechopen.70833

Different formulations, including silicone- and petroleum-based products (such as vaseline), are applied by burns units around the world with their selection appearing to be based on historical practice, clinical experience, and because patients have confidence in such treatments [36].

Although the need for scar tissue hydration is supported by almost all researches because of the enhanced transepidermal water loss rates compared to healthy skin, information and literature on the ideal composition of moisturizers for burn scar treatment are quite limited [24].

2.4. Ultrasound

Tissues with high collagen content such as scar tissue show a high attenuation for ultrasound energy. It has been reported that topical therapeutic ultrasound application to scar tissue causes a temperature rise in scar tissue, which provides an increase in the elasticity of collagen and thus enlarges the range of motion. It is also declared that application of topical ultrasound improves the pain seen in scars [24, 37–39].

But, in their randomized placebo controlled double blind study, with a low overall bias rating score, Ward et al. found no significant intergroup results on range of motion and pain [37].

2.5. Electroacupuncture

Cuignet et al. designed a study to observe the effects of a combination of manual (MA) and electro-acupuncture (EA) on the pain scores and on the sensory thresholds of the nociceptive pathways in patients presenting with pathological burn scars (PPBS). And, at the end of the study, they demonstrated that EA combined to MA reduces the pain scores of patients suffering from pain associated with burn scar. Using quantitative sensory testing (QST), they confirmed that the pain of PPBS comes from a peripheral hyperalgesia eliminated by E/MA. And, they also observed a significant relief of pruritus after E/MA [40].

2.6. Onion extract

It was reported that, in a study with 120 Asian patients, onion extract decreased the rate of scar formation in dark-skinned patients receiving laser treatment of tattoos, and the enhancement in width of scar after thoracic surgery was less for onion extract-treated fresh scars than in untreated scars after 1 year of treatment. On the other hand, in a side-by-side, randomized, double-blinded, split-scar study, scar cosmesis or symptomatology did not show any improvements with application of onion extract gel, when compared with standard therapy in the management of postoperative wounds [41, 42]. It is thought that the effect of onion extract therapy on decrease in scar height may increase when used with occlusive silicone dressing [43]. In a randomized controlled trial with 60 patients of median sternotomy, the combination of onion extract and silicone products was seen effective in the prevention of hypertrophic scar formation. Onion extract is also effective in burn scars. It was observed that combination of onion extract and silicone gel provided good results in 45 patients with postburn hypertrophic scar [44, 45].

2.7. Massage therapy

Hypertrophic scar development is a common complication after burn injury and the incidence is up to 77%. The existence of hypertrophic scar after a burn trauma may lead to many physical and psychological impairments, including pruritus, increased pain levels, scar contracture and limited ROM, elevated anxiety levels, and decreased health-related quality of life [46].

Massage therapy is a non-surgical conservative method that is used to reduce the negative results of hypertrophic scar after burn injuries [47]. The aim of massage therapy is to produce relaxation, reduce the pain, or improve circulation with the manipulation of the skin and underlying tissues with varying degrees of hand pressure. Classical massage consists of movements such as petrissage (kneading), effleurage (stroking and gliding), and tapotement (percussion). But, in different burn rehabilitation centers, many kinds of massage techniques are applied [47, 48].

Scar massage has various positive clinical utilities in scar management including decreased scar thickness, decreased pruritus, decreased pain and skin sensitivity, increased scar pliability and range of movement, and decreased anxiety [46].

Severe itching/pruritus is a common complication after burn injuries, especially in patients who have wounds on leg and arm, and the incidence in adult patients is up to 87%. Itching is not just itching and usually associated with disruption of daily living activities, anxiety and sleep disturbance. Pain is another common complication after burn trauma. Pain and related conditions such as depression and anxiety may influence the wound healing process and consequently adversely affects the patient's functioning. In patients who have been exposed to burn trauma, alternative or complementary treatments may be beneficial in the decrease of itching or pain, and these applications are not widely used. The research has shown that massage therapy reduces various types of pain [49].

A possible mechanism of the pain relief effect of the touch may be through the gate theory. Gate theory expresses that pain can be relieved by pressure or cold application. Since receptor fibers-related pressure and cold stimuli are larger and more myelinated, they reach the brain receptors more rapidly and close the gate before the smaller, less myelinated pain fibers reach the brain receptors. Massage therapy has been also showed to lessen anxiety and stress hormone levels in burn patients and provides an improvement in redness, pruritus, lichenification, scaling, and excoriation. Increased vagal activity, which may enhance more relaxation and decrease the peripheral vasoconstriction associated with sympathetic activity, provided by massage therapy may be the potential mechanism for reducing stress and improving other skin findings mentioned above [49].

Additionally, it is showed that massage therapy has some mechanical effects associated with an improvement in venous return and lymphatic drainage. Moreover, massage therapy stimulates movement between muscle fibers, which results in more fluid muscle movement. In their randomized controlled trial, Cho et al. reported that massage therapy affects the scar thickness, scar elasticity, scar melanin and erythema, and scar transepidermal water loss (TEWL) positively as well as reducing pain and itching [50].

In summary, findings from studies show that scar massage is effective in improving scar height, vascularity, pliability, pain, pruritus, and depression in patients with hypertrophic scarring as a result of burn injury [46–50].

2.8. Combined therapy

Among the conservative therapies, the most common options used as a combination treatment for burn scars are pressure therapy and silicone gel therapy. Since the mechanisms of action of silicone gels and pressure therapy are complementary to each other, it appeared to be evident that the combined therapy of silicone and pressure would give mixed and more effective results [24].

Pressure therapy has been used since the early 1970s as a conservative method in hypertrophic scar prevention or treatment and usually applied in the forms of garment or dressing. It was reported that pressure therapy has potential to prevent hypertrophic scar formation or limited its maturation and consequently to provide a better appearance of scars. Pressure therapy can reduce itching and pain as well as improve the appearance of scars.

Although how pressure therapy prevents the formation or maturation of hypertrophic scar has not yet been fully elucidated, the pressure caused by the pressure garments which is thought to reduce blood flow, oxygen, and nutrient support to the scar tissue can diminish collagen synthesis. Because of the mechanical load effect of the pressure therapy on the scar zone also leads to the rearrangement of the collagen fibers, thickness of scar tends to reduce and scar tissue becomes more pliable [18, 22, 24].

Silicone gels have been used as a conservative method in the treatment of hypertrophic scar since 1980. It is thought that silicone gels diminish evaporation, provide a better homeostasis, reduce edema and vasodilatation, inhibit activity of mast cells, prevent excessive extracellular matrix formation, form a pressure on scar zone, and hydrate the scar tissue [26, 51].

In some previous studies, it was showed that combination of pressure therapy and silicone gel therapy is more effective in reduction of scar thickness, pliability, pigmentation, pain, and pruritus than the use of these treatments alone. Furthermore, it was reported that combination therapy provided an earlier response to these scar parameters. On the other hand, in some other studies, no significant different results were found between combination and non-combination groups [51, 52].

The general view is that combined treatment with both pressure therapy and silicone gels should be implemented on hypertrophic scar to enhance the effectiveness of treatments and reduce the duration needed for treatment [51].

Author details

Mehmet Unal

Address all correspondence to: dr.munal1101@gmail.com

Faculty of Medicine, Department of Dermatology and Venereology, Selcuk University, Konya, Turkey

References

[1] Alhady SM, Sivanantharajah K. Keloids in various races. A review of 175 cases. Plastic and Reconstructive Surgery. 1969;**44**(6):564-566

[2] Niessen FB, Spauwen PH, Schalkwijk J, Kon M. On the nature of hypertrophic scars and keloids: A review. Plastic and Reconstructive Surgery. 1999;**104**(5):1435-1458

[3] Marneros AG, Norris JE, Olsen BR, Reichenberger E. Clinical genetics of familial keloids. Archives of Dermatology. 2001;**137**(11):1429-1434

[4] Smith P, Mosiello G, Deluca L, Ko F, Maggi S, Robson MC. TGF-beta2 activates proliferative scar fibroblasts. The Journal of Surgical Research. 1999;**82**(2):319-323

[5] Ehrlich HP, Desmoulière A, Diegelmann RF, Cohen IK, Compton CC, Garner WL, Kapanci Y, Gabbiani G. Morphological and immunochemical differences between keloid and hypertrophic scar. The American Journal of Pathology. 1994;**145**(1):105-113

[6] Candy LH, Cecilia LT, Ping ZY. Effect of different pressure magnitudes on hypertrophic scar in a Chinese population. Burns. 2010;**36**(8):1234-1241

[7] Armour A, Scott GP, Tredget EE. Cellular and molecular pathology of HTS: Basis for treatment. Wound Repair and Regeneration. 2000;**15**:6-17

[8] Tejero-Trujeque R. How do fibroblasts interact with the extracellular matrix in wound contraction? Journal of Wound Care. 2000;**10**:237-242

[9] Leblebici MHF, Akman M, Noyan T, Tarim A, Bagis S, Adam M. Quality of life after burn injury: The impact of joint contracture. Burns. 2007;**33**:47

[10] Rumsey N, White P. Exploring the psychosocial concerns of out-patients with disfiguring conditions. Journal of Wound Care. 2003;**12**:247-252

[11] Van den Kerckhove E, Stappaerts K, Fieuws S, Laperre J, Massage P, Flour M, Boeckx W. The assessment of erythema and thickness on burn related scars during pressure garmenttherapy as preventive measure for hypertrophic scarring. Burns. 2005;**31**(6):696-702

[12] The Scar Information Service. What is a scar? Available from: http://www.scarinfo.org [Retrieved September 4, 2007]

[13] Engrav LH, Heimbach DM, Rivara FP, Moore ML, Wang J, Carrougher GJ, Costa B, Numhom S, Calderon J, Gibran NS. 12-year within-wound study of the effectiveness of custom pressure garment therapy. Burns. 2010;**36**(7):975-983

[14] Staley MJ, Richard RL. Use of pressure to treat hypertrophic burn scars. Advances in Wound Care. 1997;**10**:44

[15] Linares HA, Larson DL, Willis-Galstaun BA. Historical notes on the use of pressure in the treatment of hypertrophic scars or keloids. Burns. 1993;**19**(1):17-21

[16] Lawrence H. Keloid (alibert) and intractable patches of chronic inflammation of the skin treated by scarification. British Medical Journal. 1898;**1**:151

[17] Larson DL, Abston S, Evans EB, Dobrkovsky M, Linares HA. Techniques for decreasing scar formation and contractures in the burned patient. The Journal of Trauma. 1971;**11**(10):807-823

[18] Ward RS. Pressure therapy for the control of hypertrophic scar formation after burn injury. The Journal of Burn Care & Rehabilitation. 1991;**12**:257-262

[19] Naismith RS. Hypertrophic scar therapy: pressure-induced remodeling and its determinants [PhD thesis]. Glasgow: University of Strathclyde; 1980

[20] Costa MAA, Peyrol S, Porto C, Comparin JPL, Foyatier LJ, Desmouliere A. Mechanical forces induce scar remodeling. American Journal of Pathology. 1999;**155**:1671-1679

[21] Hosoda GH, Holloway GA, Heimbach DM. Laser doppler flowmetry for the early detection of hypertrophic burn scars. Journal of Burn Care and Rehabilitation. 1986;**7**:496-497

[22] Leung KS, Sher A, Clark JA, Cheng CYJ, Leung PC. Microcirculation in hypertrophic scar after burn injury. Journal of Burn Care and Rehabilitation. 1989;**10**:436-444

[23] Clark JA, Leung KS, Cheng JCY, Leung PC. The hypertrophic scar and microcirculation properties. Burns. 1996;**22**:447-450

[24] Anthonissen M, Daly D, Janssens T, Van den Kerckhove E. The effects of conservative treatments on burn scars: A systematic review. Burns. 2016;**42**(3):508-518

[25] Ng SFF. Medical clothing: The stress relaxation and shrinkage of pressure garments. International Journal of Clothing Science and Technology. 1994;**6**:17-27

[26] Momeni M, Hafezi F, Rahbar H, Karimi H. Effects of silicone gel on burn scars. Burns. 2009;**35**(1):70-74

[27] Van der Wal M, van Zuijlen P, van de Ven P, Middelkoop E. Topical silicone gel versus placebo in promoting the maturation of burn scars: A randomized controlled trial. Plastic and Reconstructive Surgery 2010;**126**:524-531

[28] Perkins K, Davey RB, Wallis KA. Silicone gel: A new treatment for burn scars and contractures. Burns, Including Thermal Injury. 1983;**9**:201-204

[29] Glenn LW. The plastic surgery educational foundation DATA committee. Silicone gel sheeting. Plastic and Reconstructive Surgery. 2001;**107**:272-275

[30] Musgrave MA, Umraw N, Gomez M, Cartotto RC. The effect of silicone gel sheets on perfusion of hypertrophic burn scars. The Journal of Burn Care & Rehabilitation. 2002;**23**:208-214

[31] Gilman TH. Silicone sheet for treatment and prevention of hypertrophic scar: A new proposal for the mechanism of efficacy. Wound Repair and Regeneration. 2003;**11**:235-236

[32] Li-Tsang CW, Lau JC, Choi J, Chan CC, Jianan L. A prospective randomized clinical trial to investigate the effect of silicone gel sheeting (Cica-care) on post-traumatic hypertrophic scar among the Chinese population. Burns. 2006;**32**(6):678-683

[33] Serghiou MA, Ott S, Farmer S, Morgan D, Gibson P, Suman OE. Comprehensive rehabilitation of the burn patient. In: Herndon D. Total Burn Care. Third ed. Philadelphia: Saunders, Elsevier Inc; 2007

[34] Suetake T, Sasai S, Zhen Y, Tagami H. Effects of silicone gel sheet on the stratum corneum hydration. British Journal of Plastic Surgery. 2000;**53**:503-507

[35] Lewis PA, Wright K, Webster A, Steer M, Rudd M, Doubrovsky A, et al. A randomized controlled pilot study comparing aqueous cream with a beeswax and herbal oil cream in the provision of relief from postburn pruritus. Journal of Burn Care & Research: Official Publication of the American Burn Association. 2012;**33**(4):e195-e200

[36] Klotz T, Kurmis R, Munn Z, Heath K, Greenwood JE. The effectiveness of moisturizers for the management of burn scars following severe burn injury: A systematic review protocol. JBI Database of Systematic Reviews and Implementation Reports. 2014;**12**:212-220

[37] Ward R, Hayes-Lundy C, Reddy R, Brockway C, Mills PJRS. Evaluation of topical therapeutic ultrasound to improve response to physical therapy and less scar contracture after burn injury. The Journal of Burn Care & Rehabilitation. 1994;**15**:74-79

[38] Bierman W. Ultrasound in the treatment of scars. Archives of Physical Medicine and Rehabilitation. 1954;**35**(4):209-214

[39] Gersten JW. Effect of ultrasound on tendon extensibility. American Journal of Physical Medicine. 1955;**34**(2):362-369

[40] Cuignet O, Pirlot A, Ortiz S, Rose T. The effects of electroacupuncture on analgesia and peripheral sensory thresholds in patientswith burn scar pain. Burns. 2015;**41**(6):1298-1305

[41] Chung VQ, Kelley L, Marra D, Jiang SB. Onion extract gel versus petrolatum emollient on new surgical scars: Prospective double-blinded study. Dermatologic Surgery. 2006;**32**:193-197

[42] Ho WS, Ying SY, Chan PC, Chan HH. Use of onion extract, heparin, allantoin gel in prevention of scarring in Chinese patients having laser removal of tattoos: A prospective randomized controlled trial. Dermatologic Surgery. 2006;**32**:891-896

[43] Hosnuter M, Payasli C, Isikdemir A, Tekerekoglu B. The effects of onion extract on hypertrophic and keloid scars. Journal of Wound Care. 2007;**16**:251-254

[44] Karagoz H, Yuksel F, Ulkur E, Evinc R. Comparison of efficacy of silicone gel, silicone gel sheeting, and topical onion extract including heparin and allantoin for the treatment of postburn hypertrophic scars. Burns. 2009;**35**:1097-1103

[45] Jeenwitheesuk K, Surakunprapha P, Jenwitheesuk K, et al. Role of silicone derivative plus onion gel extract in presternal hypertrophic scar protection: A prospective randomized,

double-blinded, controlled trial. International Wound Journal. 2012;**9**:397-402. E-published ahead of print December 14, 2011

[46] Ault P, Plaza A, Paratz J. Scar massage for hypertrophic burns scarring-systematic review. Burns. 2017 pii: S0305-4179(17)30296-6

[47] Roques C. Massage applied to scars. Wound Repair and Regeneration. 2002;**10**(2):126-128

[48] Roh YS, Cho H, Oh JO, Yoon CJ. Effects of skin rehabilitation massage therapy on pruritus, skin status, and depression in burn survivors. Taehan Kanho Hakhoe Chi. 2007;**37**(2):221-226

[49] Field T, Peck M, Hernandez-Reif M, Krugman S, Burman I, Ozment-Schenck L. Postburn itching, pain and psychological symptoms are reduced with massage therapy. The Journal of Burn Care & Rehabilitation. 2000;**21**:189-193

[50] Cho YS, Jeon JH, Hong A, Yang HT, Yim H, Cho YS, et al. The effect of burn rehabilitation massage therapy on hypertrophic scar after burn: A randomized controlled trial. Burns. 2014 Dec;**40**(8):1513-1520

[51] Li-Tsang CWP, Zheng YP, Lau JC. A randomized clinical trial to study the effect of silicone gel dressing and pressure therapy on posttraumatic hypertrophic scars. Journal of Burn Care & Research. 2010;**31**:448-457

[52] Harte D, Gordon J, Shaw M, Stinson M, Porter-Armstrong A. The use of pressure and silicone in hypertrophic scar management in burns patients: A pilot randomized controlled trial. Journal of Burn Care & Research. 2009;**30**:632-642

Chapter 5

Herbal Therapy for Burns and Burn Scars

Serap Maden, Emel Erdal Çalıkoğlu and
Pertevniyal Bodamyalızade

Additional information is available at the end of the chapter

http://dx.doi.org/10.5772/intechopen.71665

Abstract

Burn wound healing is a complex process including inflammation, epithelialization, granulation, neovascularization, and wound contraction. Modern therapies present a large number of options, while traditional therapies are promising effective choices. Plant-based products have been used in the treatment of wounds for centuries worldwide. Recently, the mechanisms behind many of these traditional therapies could be explained in detail. The most commonly found mechanisms behind the herbal source products supporting wound healing are mostly their antioxidant, anti-inflammatory, antimicrobial, cell proliferative, and angiogenic effects. However there is not much more studies demonstrated in patients except *Aloe vera* and *Avena* sp., herbal treatment still show a lot of promise in the future. It is important not to ignore possible toxic and allergic effects of plants and phytochemical agents, but the studies mostly resulted with antitoxic effects. Several herbs show efficient results with therapies of wounds also in burn wounds, which may be considered as an option for treatment. On the other hand, herbal treatment in burn wounds still needs to have more clinical and pharmaceutical studies to place in modern therapies safely.

Keywords: burn wound, herbal therapy, plant, phytochemical, wound healing

1. Introduction

Skin is the largest organ of the human body that protects the internal organs from the external environment and prevents body dehydration. It can be traumatized by burn injuries, chronic wounds, excision, tumors, and other dermatological conditions [1]. Burns are one of the most commonly seen trauma incidents and burn wounds need a meticulous care for progress, which causes major medical and economic costs [2]. Burns have extensive categories that may result from heat, cold, chemical, or radiation exposure causing acute cutaneous wounds [3]. Burn wounds are classified into three subgroups according to the depth as first degree (superficial), second degree (partial thickness), and third degree (full thickness) [4]. Process of the wound healing has complicated pathways that do not occur in a linear way and can progress forward or backward during the phases depending on various intrinsic and extrinsic factors [5]. After the cutaneous injury, hemostasis is achieved with the activation of platelets resulting in clot formation, which essentially acts as a temporary wound closure mechanism [6]. Burn wound healing is a complex process including inflammation due to the disruption of blood vessels and extravasation of blood constituents, reepithelialization, formation of granulation tissue handled by macrophages and fibroblasts that are responsible for the recovery of the extracellular matrix (ECM), neovascularization as well as migration and mitogenic stimulation of endothelial cells and wound contraction as a result of the interaction between cells, ECM, and cytokines [7]. Neutrophils begin placing to the injury area within hours of the injury, by the effects of platelet-derived growth factors (PDGF), transforming growth factor-beta (TGF-B), and fibroblast growth factor (FGF), that are potent chemotactic agents for neutrophils [6].

Several biochemicals are involved in burn healing process including matrix metalloproteinases, superoxide dismutase, catalase, reduced glutathione, malondialdehyde, myeloperoxidase, vascular endothelial growth factor, hydroxyproline, hexosamine, ascorbic acid (vitamin C) and protein content in damaged and surrounding tissue, serum levels of aspartate transaminase, alanine transaminase, lactate dehydrogenase, blood urea nitrogen, creatinine as indicators of liver and kidney damage, and tumor necrosis factor (TNF) for the evaluation of generalized tissue damage [8]. Moreover, wound repair process has also a chronic progression because of oxygen free radicals. Oxidative stress causes delay in healing and concludes with secondary tissue damage. It is assumed that antioxidant therapy may have a defense effect by decreasing free oxygen radicals and strengthening cellular antioxidant mechanisms, which supports the healing process of the wound [9]. Consequently, compounds playing roles as free-radical neutralizers that include antimicrobial properties may have an important effect in enhancing wound healing. Several traditional herbal-based therapies have been shown to possess antioxidant activity and also enhance wound healing in in vitro studies [10].

Excessive tissue growing may result with aberrant patterns of wounds. Hypertrophic scars and keloids are deviant form results of wound healing that are also seen after burn wounds. Aberrant function of fibroblasts and exaggerate accumulation of ECM during wound healing with a dysregulated response to cutaneous injuries, result in an excessive deposition of collagen. Hypertrophic scars have a raised and firm surface with red or pink in color and usually limited to wound area, while keloids have raised firm and irregular surface usually dark red and pigmented in color that extends into the neighboring skin. Keloids are tougher lesions to treat because of not regressing, also difficult to manage surgically, that do not provoke scar contractures with time, contrary to hypertrophic scars [11, 12]. There are plant-based agents that may inhibit nuclear factor κB (NF-κB) and TGF-β1 signaling in keloid fibroblasts and also decrease ECM production [3].

Various wound care products are used for the management of scars, like autografts and allografts, creams and solutions, wound dressings and alternative tissue-engineered skin substitutes [1]. In recent years, a variety of commercially available wound dressings were launched. However, they possess certain critical limitations such as addition of antimicrobial agents, which might include cytotoxic effects, especially on prolonged treatment period, causing to delay wound healing. Some of the marketed dressings lose their moisturizing effect, which makes them adhere to the surface of the wound and damage the newly formed epithelium [13]. After burn damage, the treatment of skin needs the use of several drugs administered separately or combined, and it is a complex and painful process [14].

In traditional medicine, there are various phytochemicals that are used for wound healing supplying enhanced healing process via anti-inflammatory or antioxidant activity [3]. However, several herbal-sourced phytochemicals have shown some efficacy in animal models on the treatment of burn wounds; only a few herb-derived phytochemicals have been studied in human trials such as *Aloe vera* and *Avena* sp. More effective natural products are being studied to get over with the side effects of chemotherapeutics [8].

2. Herbal therapies

2.1. *Aloe vera*

Extensive study results showed that herbs especially *A. vera* has an effective anti-inflammatory and wound healing effect. *A. vera* belongs to the Liliaceal family, which is a perennial succulent plant [15]. It origins from South Africa, widely used in conventional therapy and of great interest for several biomedical, pharmaceutical, and cosmetic applications [1]. Studies are mostly about the anti-inflammatory and wound healing effects. The gel form of *A. vera* has demonstrated the progress in wound, burn, and frostbite healing, showing known as anti-inflammatory effects also antifungal, hypoglycemic, and gastroprotective effects [15]. Furthermore, due to the features of *A. vera* as anti-inflammatory, antibacterial, antiseptic, and its reliability to inducing collagen synthesis during the wound healing, its gel form is thought to be used for the treatment of skin disorders [1]. *A. vera* has an analgesic effect and also been used in a host of curative purposes including treatment of skin disorders and healing of wounds [16]. *A. vera* gel has a significant effect that improves the synthesis of collagen and the degree of collagen cross-linking, after topical and systemic administration in wounds created in a diabetic rat model. Also, it is mentioned that the oral administration of *A. vera* significantly induces the proliferation of fibroblasts, the collagen deposition, and angiogenesis in radiation-exposed rats [17].

A. vera is a choice for treating burns because the colorless gel that comes from the leaf parenchyma is a potent moisturizing agent; it also helps in the healing process of skin lesions and alleviates pain [16, 18]. In a review, no withdrawal or serious adverse reaction was reported. The unwanted symptoms reported were only irritation, itching, discomfort, and minimal transient pain; on the other hand, these symptoms were common signs in burns, and they were found in both the *A. vera* and the control groups. Contamination with anthraquinone while using topical fresh *A. vera* has a potential cause of the irritation [19]. The polymer film formulation containing hyaluronate and alginate appears to be a promising approach for the application of substances, able to reduce damage and facilitate the healing process, like *A. vera* extracts and the antioxidant vitamin E acetate [16]. Burn healing and anti-inflammatory activity was observed in topical treatment with *A. vera* gel preparations [20]. A study of human demonstrated the efficacy of *A. vera* on second-degree burn wound patients [21–23]. In a study, it was reported that TNF-a, interleukin-6 (IL-6), and leukocyte adhesion were found to be decreased in a rat model of burn wound treated with *A. vera* gel. It was also showed to be an antibacterial effect against *Klebsiella pneumoniae*, a nosocomial pathogen in another study [8].

2.2. Curcumin

Curcumin is a polyphenol compound, diferuloylmethane, responsible for the yellow pigmentation. Curcumin is a chemical compound present in the Asian spice named turmeric or *Curcuma longa*. It is used in Indian and Chinese cuisine; also, it has been used topically for cutaneous wounds including ulcers, traditionally in the Indian subcontinent [24, 25]. It has antiproliferative, anti-invasive, and antiangiogenic effects; also, it is a therapeutic agent in wound healing. Curcumin-incorporated collagen sheets were designed for dermal wound healing. These membranes supply higher antioxidant activity, hydrothermal stability, and faster wound reduction compared to collagen-treated wounds. For effective infection control, curcumin-included membranes could be used by means of prolonged antimicrobial activity [15]. Curcumin is a phytochemical candidate for the treatment of hyperinflammatory burn wounds by the mechanism of suppression of TNF-a and IL-1 production by human macrophages anti-inflammatory properties [3].

In hypertrophic scarring and keloids, there is an abundance of TGF-B1 expression, fibroblast proliferation, and excess collagen and ECM synthesis [26]. In scleroderma, which is another fibrotic skin disease, curcumin has also been shown to inhibit TGF-B1 signaling [27]. Curcumin is a potent inhibitor of NF-κB, inhibits TGF-B1 signaling in keloid fibroblasts, and also decreases ECM production [3]. In vitro, it is showed that curcumin also suppresses the proliferation cascades of keloids and hypertrophic scar-acquired fibroblasts [28].

2.3. Honey

Honey is a nutritious thick carbohydrate-rich syrup, which was effectively known and used since ancient times in traditional medicine. Today, honey has a broad area being used due to its evidenced therapeutic effects. It is a well-known antibacterial, antiparasitic, pain reliever, and it has proven efficient against respiratory tract infections [13]. Honey has been used as a topical treatment for chronic wounds and burns in traditional medicine by diverse parts around the globe [29]. It has been used for burns in various ancient societies such as Greek and Roman physicians, and also for the treatment of burn wounds [30]. It was shown in a study that Leptospermum honey was potently active against antibiotic-resistant clinical pathogens [31]. Antibacterial features of honey are about its high osmolarity, low pH, and hydrogen peroxide production that accelerate the wound healing process [13]. Since chronic wounds and burns are particularly vulnerable to infections, honey's antibacterial effect attracts to be a therapy method [3]. The phytochemical components, such as flavonoids and phenolic acids, act as antioxidants due to their free radical removing activities, which save cells from the damage due to free oxygen radicals and decrease the inflammatory response [13]. Its immunomodulatory effects are useful for the management of chronic wounds. Honey is also shown to promote angiogenesis and fibroblast proliferation in human clinical trials [3]. It is shown in rat models of partial-thickness burn injuries, honey usage shortened the period of epithelialization and increased wound contraction compared to vehicle controls [32]. Honey carries protease enzymes that help debridement cleaning out of the wounds [33]. Honey overcomes the hyperinflammatory microenvironment on chronic wounds via its anti-inflammatory effects by the inhibition of cyclooxygenase-2 (COX-2), inducible nitric oxide synthase (iNOS), TNF-a, and IL-6 expression [34]. Also honey contains various compounds including flavonoids, phenolic acids, catalase, peroxidase, carotenoids, and ascorbic acid, which possess antioxidant properties that can neutralize the abundance of free radicals found in chronic wounds [35, 36].

Using honey over burned area supplies an advantage of wetter environment. It saves the burned surface entirety; also, it is nonadherent and provides a bacterial barrier that prevents cross infection and prevents infecting bacteria [13]. In a systematic review of randomized controlled trials of eight studies in humans comparing the efficacy of honey to silver sulfadiazine-impregnated gauze demonstrated that honey had a superior healing effect, yet burn characteristics were limited to superficial and partial thickness only [37]. Honey debrides the wound, inhibits scar formation, and induces wound healing by stimulating tissue regeneration process so that it reduces the need for skin grafting. There are no adverse effects reported from using honey in burn healing [13]. Honey also has been shown to be protective against hypertrophic scarring as a result of burn wounds. In a randomized controlled trial, the effects of honey were compared to silver sulfadiazine in 104 patients with superficial burns. Hypertrophic scarring and postburn contracture in the honey-treated group have significantly lower incidence in comparison to the silver sulfadiazine-treated group [38].

2.4. *Terminalia* genus

Some *Terminalia* species have been reported to have wound-healing properties, antioxidant and antimicrobial activity with anti-inflammatory effects. *Terminalia chebula* extract, chebulagic acid (CA), is an antioxidant compound, when cultured with macrophages in vitro, significantly suppressed NF-B activation as well as TNF-a and COX-2 expression. These results show the possibility of topical application of *T. chebula* that would be beneficial in hyperinflammatory wounds such as chronic diabetic wounds or burns. In burn wounds, the extracts of *T. chebula* accelerate wound healing in comparison to 1% silver sulfadiazine in rat models [39, 40]. *Terminalia sericea* antimicrobial activity against *Staphylococcus aureus*, *Streptococcus pyogenes*, and *Pseudomonas aeruginosa* has also been reported [3].

2.5. *Avena* sp.

Avena sp. used in shower and bath oil containing 5% colloidal oat meal in patients with partial-thickness burn showed significant decreasing in itch in comparison with control group [41].

2.6. *Zanthoxylum bungeanum*

Z. bungeanum maxim seed oil (ZBSO) was found to be effective in wound-healing activity on experimentally burned rats. It is thought to be the increased antioxidant activity as evidenced by the increase in superoxide dismutase level and decrease in malondialdehyde level, anti-inflammatory action through NF-κB signaling pathway, and accelerated collagen synthesis through the decrease of Matrix metalloproteinase-2 and Matrix metalloproteinase-9 expressions. These effects of ZBSO might result with the early reepithelialization and faster wound closure [2].

2.7. *Hippophae rhamnoides*

Oral and topical administration of *H. rhamnoides* seed oil showed progression in tissue regeneration, matrix metalloproteinase (MMP) 2 and 9, vascular endothelial growth factor (VEGF), collagen type-III, DNA, total protein, hydroxyproline and hexosamine content in the granulation tissues, as well as decrease in reactive oxygen species and edema. Omega 3 and omega 6 fatty acids, tocopherols, and carotenoids are probable active components of the oil [42]. Moreover, the leaves of *H. rhamnoides* were showed in vivo burn healing effect by increasing epithelialization, MMP-2 and 9, VEGF, hydroxyproline, hexosamine, collagen type-III, and antioxidant function. In vitro study in chick chorioallantoic membrane also demonstrated the angiogenic effect of the plant extract [43].

2.8. *Calotropis procera* Aiton

C. procera Aiton, named as *Calotropis*, is native to South-west and South-East Asia and Africa and also grows in the Caribbean Islands, in Central and South America. *Calotropis'* latex contains tannins known to advance wound healing with their astringent and antimicrobial properties providing wound contraction and increased rate of epithelialization. In complementary and alternative medicine, the whole plant of *Calotropis*, leaves, barks, and its latex have been employed in the treatment and management of many health conditions for dressing fresh skin burns. In a trial study with rabbits, *Calotropis* latex was shown to have dual effects on wound healing. It induces florid granulation tissues, inhibiting exaggerated response of fibroblasts and aberrant collagens in the matrix that might be supportive of its potential antikeloidal activity. It is demonstrated that reduction in the quantity and width of the broad band collagens in the group treated with *Calotropis* latex means in collagen is inhibited by *Calotropis'* latex. The result of this study suggests that *Calotropis'* latex can be a potential source of therapeutic agents that can be used in the treatment of keloid [11].

2.9. *Punica granatum*

P. granatum L., is also known as pomegranate. In Traditional Chinese and Indian Medicine, it is used for traumatic hemorrhage, ulcers, nose bleeds, and aphthae. The therapeutic properties of pomegranate include ellagitannins represented by ellagic acid (EA), gallic acid, and punicalagin. Mo et al. showed that in an antioxidant assay-guided extraction of pomegranate peel, ellagic acid (EA) was found to be the marker compound and major antioxidant. It was found to be in vitro and in vivo anti-inflammatory activities. *P. granatum* is a potential antioxidant therapy for burn wound healing [44, 45].

2.10. *Chromolaena odorata*

C. odorata is a plant in southern Asia and western Africa, and has been traditionally used for the treatment of wounds in Vietnam for many years [3]. *C. odorata* presents its wound healing property using multiple mechanisms. The extract of *C. odorata* contains many antioxidant compounds that progress wound healing process. It reduces the bleeding and clotting time as the first-line function of wound healing. It also has an anti-inflammatory effect that provides protection for the cells from destruction. *C. odorata* has antibacterial activities against both gram-positive and gram-negative bacteria, suggesting that it may reduce the wound infections [46]. It has been shown that *C. odorata* promotes wound contraction in in vitro models, and also promotes fibroblast proliferation. Moreover, *C. odorata* has been demonstrated to have protective effects on human fibroblasts and keratinocytes against the oxidative damage of hydrogen peroxide [3].

Herbal therapies	Healing mechanisms in burn wounds
A. vera	Anti-inflammatory [1, 15] Antibacterial [1] Antifungal [15] Analgesic [16] Antikeloidal effect [17]
Curcumin	Antiproliferative, antiangiogenic [15] Antikeloidal effect [28]
Honey	Antibacterial, antiparasitic, analgesic, antioxidant [13] Immunomodulatory effect [3] Antikeloidal effect [38]
Terminalia genus	Anti-inflammatory [39] Antibacterial [3]
Avena sp.	Antipruritic [41]
Zanthoxylum bungeanum	Antioxidant [2]
Hippophae rhamnoides	Antioxidant [42, 43]
Calotropis	Antibacterial, antikeloidal effect [11]
Punica granatum	Antioxidant, anti-inflammatory [44, 45]
Chromolaena odorata	Antioxidant [3, 46] Anti-inflammatory, antibacterial [39, 46]
Centella asiatica	Increasing reepithelialization and keratinization [47]

Table 1. Healing mechanisms in burn wounds of herbal therapies.

2.11. *Centella asiatica*

C. asiatica extracts of aerial parts were investigated for burn wound healing activity, and being the most potent one, ethylacetate extract, also all types of the extracts had positive effect on wound healing by increasing reepithelialization and keratinization [47]. *C. asiatica* extracts, madecassoside, and asiaticoside and their corresponding aglycones (madecassic acid and asiatic acid) isolated from were shown to be stimulatory action on synthesis of collagen type I and III by activating fibroblasts via TGF-B in human skin fibroblast cells. Moreover, wound contraction in mice was demonstrated by means of madecassoside and asiaticoside [48]. Oral administration of madecassoside increased proliferation of fibroblasts and granulation tissue, hydroxyproline content, collagen synthesis, and angiogenesis in burn wounds of ICR mice [49] (**Table 1**).

3. Other herbal sources of burn wound care

Ficus asperifolia, Bridelia ferruginea, Gossypium arboreum [3], *Cucurbita moschata* [50], *Linum usitatissimum* L. [51], *Sesamum indicum* L., *Pistacia atlantica* Desf., *Cannabis sativa* L., *Juglans regia* L. [52], *Scutellariae* (altissimae, galericulatae, hastifoliae) [53].

Author details

Serap Maden*, Emel Erdal Çalıkoğlu and Pertevniyal Bodamyalızade

*Address all correspondence to: madenser@gmail.com

Department of Dermatology and Venereology, Near East University School of Medicine, Nicosia, Cyprus

References

[1] Pereira RF, Carvalho A, Gil MH, Mendes A, Bártolo PJ. Influence of *Aloe vera* on water absorption and enzymatic in vitro degradation of alginate hydrogel films. Carbohydrate Polymers. 2013;**98**:311-320. DOI: 10.1016/j.carbpol.2013.05.076

[2] Li XQ, Kang R, Huo JC, Xie YH, Wang SW, Cao W. Wound-healing activity of *Zanthoxylum bungeanum* maxim seed oil on experimentally burned rats. Pharmacognosy Magazine. 2017;**13**:363-371. DOI: 10.4103/pm. pm_211_16

[3] Shah A, Amini-Nik S. The role of phytochemicals in the inflammatory phase of wound healing. International Journal of Molecular Sciences. 2017;**18**. pii: E1068. DOI: 10.3390/ijms18051068

[4] Dumville JC, Munson C. Negative pressure wound therapy for partial-thickness burns. Cochrane Database of Systematic Reviews. 2012;**12**:CD006215. DOI: 10.1002/14651858.CD006215.pub3

[5] Wild T, Rahbarnia A, Kellner M, Sobotka L, Eberlein T. Basics in nutrition and wound healing. Nutrition. 2010;**26**:862-866. DOI: 10.1016/j.nut.2010.05.008

[6] Portou MJ, Baker D, Abraham D, Tsui J. The innate immune system, toll-like receptors and dermal wound healing: A review. Vascular Pharmacology. 2015;**71**:31-36. DOI: 10.1016/j.vph.2015.02.007

[7] Guo S, Dipietro LA. Factors affecting wound healing. Journal of Dental Research. 2010;**89**:219-229. DOI: 10.1177/0022034509359125

[8] Bahramsoltani R, Farzaei MH, Rahimi R. Medicinal plants and their natural components as future drugs for the treatment of burn wounds: An integrative review. Archives of Dermatological Research. 2014;**306**:601-617. DOI: 10.1007/s00403-014-1474-6

[9] Parihar A, Parihar MS, Milner S, Bhat S. Oxidative stress and anti-oxidative mobilization in burn injury. Burns. 2008;**34**(1):6-17. DOI: 10.1016/j.burns.2007.04.009

[10] Suntar I, Akkol E, Nahar L, Sarker S. Wound healing and antioxidant properties: Do they coexist in plants? Free Radicals and Antioxidants 2012;**2**:1-7. DOI: 10.5530/ax.2012.2.1

[11] Aderounmu AO, Omonisi AE, Akingbasote JA, Makanjuola M, Bejide RA, Orafidiya LO, Adelusola KA. Wound-healing and potential anti-keloidal properties of the latex of *Calotropis procera* (Aiton) Asclepiadaceae in rabbits. African Journal of Traditional, Complementary, and Alternative Medicines. 2013;**10**:574-579

[12] Hsu YC, Chen MJ, Yu YM, Ko SY, Chang CC. Suppression of TGF β1/smad pathway and extracellular matrix production in primary keloid fibroblasts by curcuminoids: Its potential therapeutic use in the chemoprevention of keloid. Archives of Dermatological Research. 2010;**302**:717-724. DOI 10.1007/s00403-010-1075-y

[13] El-Kased RF, Amer RI, Attia D, Elmazar MM. Honey-based hydrogel: In vitro and comparative in vivo evaluation for burn wound healing. Scientific Reports. 2017;**7**:9692. DOI: 10.1038/s41598-017-08771-8

[14] Drago H, Marín GH, Sturla F, Roque G, Mártire K, Díaz Aquino V, Lamonega R, Gardiner C, Ichim T, Riordan N, Raimondi JC, Bossi S, Samadikuchaksaraei A, van Leeuwen M, Tau JM, Núñez L, Larsen G, Spretz R, Mansilla E. The next generation of burns treatment: Intelligent films and matrix, controlled enzymatic debridement, and adult stem cells. Transplantation Proceedings. 2010;**42**:345-349. DOI: 10.1016/j.transproceed.2009.11.031

[15] Tummalapalli M, Berthet M, Verrier B, Deopura BL, Alam MS, Gupta B. Composite wound dressings of pectin and gelatin with *Aloe vera* and curcumin as bioactive agents. International Journal of Biological Macromolecules. 2016;**82**:104-113. DOI: 10.1016/j.ijbiomac.2015.10.087

[16] Pereira GG, Guterres SS, Balducci AG, Colombo P, Sonvico F. Polymeric films loaded with vitamin E and *Aloe vera* for topical application in the treatment of burn wounds. BioMed Research International. 2014;**2014**:641590. DOI: 10.1155/2014/641590

[17] Atiba A, Ueno H, Uzuka Y. The effect of *Aloe vera* oral administration on cutaneous wound healing in type 2 diabetic rats. The Journal of Veterinary Medical Science. 2011; **73**:583-589. DOI: 10.1292/jvms.10-0438

[18] Cuttle L, Kempf M, Kravchuk O, et al. The efficacy of *Aloe vera*, tea tree oil and saliva as first aid treatment for partial thickness burn injuries. Burns. 2008;**34**:1176-1182

[19] Maenthaisong R, Chaiyakunapruk N, Niruntraporn S, Kongkaew C. The efficacy of *Aloe vera* used for burn wound healing: A systematic review. Burns. 2007;**33**(6):713-718

[20] Hajhashemi V, Ghannadi A, Heidari AH. Anti-inflammatory and wound healing activities of *Aloe littoralis* in rats. Research in Pharmaceutical Sciences. 2012;**7**:73-78

[21] Shahzad MN, Ahmed N. Effectiveness of *Aloe vera* gel compared with 1% silver sulphadiazine cream as burn wound dressing in second degree burns. The Journal of the Pakistan Medical Association. 2013;**63**:225-230

[22] Duansak D, Somboonwong J, Patumraj S. Effects of Aloe vera on leukocyte adhesion and TNF-alpha and IL-6 levels in burn wounded rats. Clinical Hemorheology and Microcirculation. 2003;**29**(3-4):239-246

[23] Kumari S, Harjai K, Chhibber S. Topical treatment of Klebsiella pneumoniae B5055 induced burn wound infection in mice using natural products. Journal of Infection in Developing Countries. 2010 Jun 30;**4**(6):367-377

[24] Biswas TK, Mukherjee B. Plant medicines of Indian origin for wound healing activity: A review. The International Journal of Lower Extremity Wounds. 2003;**2**:25-39. DOI: 10.1177/1534734603002001006

[25] Chan MM. Inhibition of tumor necrosis factor by curcumin, a phytochemical. Biochemical Pharmacology. 1995;**49**:1551-1556

[26] Arno AI, Amini-Nik S, Blit PH, Al-Shehab M, Belo C, Herer E, Jeschke MG. Effect of human Wharton's jelly mesenchymal stem cell paracrine signaling on keloid fibroblasts. Stem Cells Translational Medicine. 2014;**3**:299-307. DOI: 10.5966/sctm.2013-0120

[27] Song K, Peng S, Sun Z, Li H, Yang R. Curcumin suppresses TGF-β signaling by inhibition of TGIF degradation in scleroderma fibroblasts. Biochemical and Biophysical Research Communications. 2011;**411**:821-825. DOI: 10.1016/j.bbrc.2011.07.044

[28] Phan TT, Sun L, Bay BH, Chan SY, Lee ST. Dietary compounds inhibit proliferation and contraction of keloid and hypertrophic scar-derived fibroblasts in vitro: Therapeutic implication for excessive scarring. The Journal of Trauma. 2003;**54**(6):1212-1224. DOI: 10.1097/01.TA.0000030630.72836.32

[29] Majtan J. Honey: An immunomodulator in wound healing. Wound Repair and Regeneration. 2014;**22**:187-192. DOI: 10.1111/wrr.12117

[30] Pećanac M, Janjić Z, Komarcević A, Pajić M, Dobanovacki D, Misković SS. Burns treatment in ancient times. Medicinski Pregled. 2013;**66**:263-267

[31] Blair SE, Cokcetin NN, Harry EJ, Carter DA. The unusual antibacterial activity of medical-grade leptospermum honey: Antibacterial spectrum, resistance and transcriptome analysis. European Journal of Clinical Microbiology & Infectious Diseases. 2009;**28**:1199-1208. DOI: 10.1007/s10096-009-0763-z

[32] Iftikhar F, Arshad M, Rasheed F, Amraiz D, Anwar P, Gulfraz M. Effects of acacia honey on wound healing in various rat models. Phytotherapy Research. 2010;**24**:583-586. DOI: 10.1002/ptr.2990

[33] Alam F, Islam MA, Gan SH, Khalil MI. Honey: A potential therapeutic agent for managing diabetic wounds. Evidence-based Complementary and Alternative Medicine. 2014; **2014**:169130. DOI: 10.1155/2014/169130

[34] Hussein SZ, Mohd Yusoff K, Makpol S, Mohd Yusof YA. Gelam honey inhibits the production of proinflammatory, mediators NO, PGE (2), TNF-α, and IL-6 in carrageenan-induced acute paw edema in rats. Evidence-based Complementary and Alternative Medicine. 2012;**2012**:109636. DOI: 10.1155/2012/109636

[35] Gheldof N, Wang XH, Engeseth NJ. Identification and quantification of antioxidant components of honeys from various floral sources. Journal of Agricultural and Food Chemistry. 2002;**50**:5870-5877. DOI: 10.1021/jf0256135

[36] Henriques A, Jackson S, Cooper R, Burton N. Free radical production and quenching in honeys with wound healing potential. The Journal of Antimicrobial Chemotherapy. 2006;**58**:773-777. DOI: 10.1093/jac/dkl336

[37] Wijesinghe M, Weatherall M, Perrin K, Beasley R. Honey in the treatment of burns: A systematic review and meta-analysis of its efficacy. The New Zealand Medical Journal. 2009;**122**:47-60

[38] Subrahmanyam M. Topical application of honey for burn wound treatment—An overview. Annals of Burns and Fire Disasters. 2007;**20**:137-139

[39] Nasiri E, Hosseinimehr SJ, Azadbakht M, Akbari J, Enayati-Fard R, Azizi S. The effect of *Terminalia chebula* extract vs. silver sulfadiazine on burn wounds in rats. Journal of Complementary & Integrative Medicine. 2015;**12**:127-135. DOI: 10.1515/jcim-2014-0068

[40] Steenkamp V, Mathivha E, Gouws MC, van Rensburg CE. Studies on antibacterial, antioxidant and fibroblast growth stimulation of wound healing remedies from South Africa. Journal of Ethnopharmacology. 2004;**95**:353-357. DOI: 10.1016/j.jep.2004.08.020

[41] Matheson JD, Clayton J, Muller MJ. The reduction of itch during burn wound healing. The Journal of Burn Care & Rehabilitation. 2001;**22**:76-81

[42] Upadhyay NK, Kumar R, Mandotra SK, Meena RN, Siddiqui MS, Sawhney RC, Gupta A. Safety and healing efficacy of sea buckthorn (*Hippophae rhamnoides* L.) seed oil on burn wounds in rats. Food and Chemical Toxicology. 2009;**47**:1146-1153. DOI: 10.1016/j.fct.2009.02.002

[43] Upadhyay NK, Kumar R, Siddiqui MS, Gupta A. Mechanism of wound-healing activity of *Hippophae rhamnoides* L. leaf extract in experimental burns. Evidence-based Complementary and Alternative Medicine. 2011;**2011**:659705. DOI: 10.1093/ecam/nep189

[44] Mo J, Panichayupakaranant P, Kaewnopparat N, Nitiruangjaras A, Reanmongkol W. Wound healing activities of standardized pomegranate rind extract and its major antioxidant ellagic acid in rat dermal wounds. Journal of Natural Medicines. 2014;**68**(2): 377-386

[45] Phan TT, Hughes MA, Cherry GW, Le TT, Pham HM. An aqueous extract of the leaves of Chromolaena odorata (formerly Eupatorium odoratum) (Eupolin) inhibits hydrated collagen lattice contraction by normal human dermal fibroblasts. Journal of Alternative and Complementary Medicine. 1996;**2**:335-343. DOI: 10.1089/act.1996.2.335

[46] Sirinthipaporn A, Jiraungkoorskul W. Wound healing property review of Siam weed, *Chromolaena odorata*. Pharmacognosy Reviews. 2017;**11**:35-38. DOI: 10.4103/phrev.phrev_53_16

[47] Somboonwong J, Kankaisre M, Tantisira B, Tantisira MH. Wound healing activities of different extracts of *Centella asiatica* in incision and burn wound models: An experimental animal study. BMC Complementary and Alternative Medicine. 2012;**12**:103. DOI: 10.1186/1472-6882-12-103

[48] Wu F, Bian D, Xia Y, Gong Z, Tan Q, Chen J, Dai Y. Identification of major active ingredients responsible for burn wound healing of *Centella asiatica* herbs. Evidence-based Complementary and Alternative Medicine. 2012;**2012**:848093. DOI: 10.1155/2012/848093

[49] Liu M, Dai Y, Li Y, Luo Y, Huang F, Gong Z, Meng Q. Madecassoside isolated from *Centella asiatica* herbs facilitates burn wound healing in mice. Planta Medica. 2008;**74**: 809-815. DOI: 10.1055/s-2008-1074533

[50] Bahramsoltani R, Farzaei MH, Abdolghaffari AH, Rahimi R, Samadi N, Heidari M, Esfandyari M, Baeeri M, Hassanzadeh G, Abdollahi M, Soltani S, Pourvaziri A, Amin G. Evaluation of phytochemicals, antioxidant and burn wound healing activities of *Cucurbita moschata* Duchesne fruit peel. Iranian Journal of Basic Medical Sciences. 2017;**20**:798-805. DOI: 10.22038/IJBMS.2017.9015

[51] Beroual K, Agabou A, Abdeldjelil MC, Boutaghane N, Haouam S, Hamdi-Pacha Y. Evaluation of crude flaxseed (*Linum usitatissimum* L) oil in burn wound healing in New Zealand rabbits. African Journal of Traditional, Complementary, and Alternative Medicines. 2017;**14**:280-286. DOI: 10.21010/ajtcam.v14i3.29

[52] Mehrabani M, Seyyedkazemi SM, Nematollahi MH, Jafari E, Mehrabani M, Mehdipour M, Sheikhshoaee Z, Mandegary A. Accelerated burn wound closure in mice with a new formula based on traditional medicine. Iranian Red Crescent Medical Journal. 2016;**18**: e26613. DOI: 10.5812/ircmj.26613

[53] Bejenaru C, Mogoşanu GD, Bejenaru LE, BiŢă A, Bălşeanu TA, Ionică FE. Effect of Scutellariae herba extracts in experimental model of skin burns: Histological and immunohistochemical assessment. Romanian Journal of Morphology and Embryology. 2016;**57**:1285-1294

Chapter 6

Platelet-Rich Plasma in Burn Treatment

Mehmet Unal

Additional information is available at the end of the chapter

http://dx.doi.org/10.5772/intechopen.70835

Abstract

As a general definition, platelet-rich plasma (PRP) is the concentration of autologous human platelets in a small amount of plasma. PRP contains important growth factors deposited in alpha-granules of platelets and plasma proteins such as fibrin, fibronectin, and vitronectin. PRP has been shown to improve wound healing process in acute trauma wounds, incisional wounds, and chronic nonhealing wounds and is a beneficial agent in reconstructions of soft and hard tissue. Furthermore, PRP enhances differentiation of epithelial cell and collagen bundle organization. Effects of growth factors in PRP on wound healing and successful results obtained with PRP treatment in other types of wound lead to the use of PRP for burn treatment.

Keywords: burn injury, wound, healing, platelet, platelet-rich plasma

1. Introduction

Platelets are small and anucleate cells derived from megakaryocytes in the bone marrow. Platelets carry vesicles containing presynthesized proteins in their granules that can be released into the local environment or transported for surface expression. Controlled and coordinated release of these factors is an important part of the normal wound healing process.

Platelet-rich plasma (PRP) is a composition comprising platelets in a plasma at a higher density than normal blood concentration. PRP has been shown to be an effective agent for bone grafting, cartilage regeneration, neovascularization, and tissue deposition in animal studies. These results have increased the interest in PRP and led to the use of PRP in human surgical applications.

PRP has been reported to be used in a wide variety of applications, mainly in problematic wound, maxillofacial, and spinal surgery. The results from these studies have provided strong evidence supporting the clinical use of PRP; however, only few include controls to clearly demonstrate the role of the PRP. Additionally, there is not a precise consensus regarding platelet-rich plasma production and characterization. This lack of consensus also prevents a standard approach in the PRP [1–9].

2. Platelets: origin, structure, distribution, and their roles in hemostasis

Platelets, discovered in the nineteenth century, are small, nucleus-free cytoplasmic cellular structures which are round or oval-shaped and have about 2 μm diameter and derived from megakaryocytes (a type of white blood cell) in the bone marrow [1]. These cellular structures were initially believed to be involved only in the hemostasis and pathological thrombus formation. Although, platelets do not have nucleus, many organelles are found in their cytoplasm including abundant mitochondria, several loops of microtubular coils giving them a robust cytoskeletal structure, and granules (alpha, delta, and lambda) [2–5].

The platelets organize the migration of cells associated with wound healing (neutrophils, macrophages, stem cells, etc.) as well as the formation of the initial clot by means of the inflammatory mediators they contain [6, 7].

Alpha granules are formed during megakaryocyte maturation, and each platelet contains approximately 50–80 alpha granules, each bound by a unit membrane [8, 9]. Alpha granules are about 200–500 nm in diameter and contain more than 30 bioactive mediators each playing a fundamental role in hemostasis and/or tissue healing. Platelets reside intravascularly and are concentrated in the spleen. The normal mean concentration of platelets in normal blood is about 140,000–400,000 platelets/mm^3. Platelets are removed by macrophages in the reticuloendothelial system after approximately 10 days in the circulation [9–11].

After tissue damage, the platelets become exposed to the damaged vessel, and these damaged vessels are places where the platelets directly contact with collagen, the basement membranes of capillaries, and subendothelial microfibrils [10]. This interaction causes the platelets to aggregate at the damaged site and change from a rounded shape to one that includes large, sticky protuberances or pseudopodia. This course is called "activation." The alpha-granules fuse with the platelet plasma membrane and release their protein contents to the surroundings during activation [11, 12].

Blood clotting begins via one of two pathways called intrinsic and extrinsic pathways [10]. The intrinsic one is started by damage or alteration to the blood, itself, whereas the extrinsic pathway is started via the contact of blood and factors that are extraneous to the blood (e.g., damaged tissue). Both cascades are associated with a series of reactions in which the inactive factors are activated. These series of reactions facilitate the formation of other mediators from precursors that go on to catalyze subsequent reactions, leading to the formation of a final clot. Although both pathways are initiated in different ways, they overlap and share common steps in the later stages of clot formation [9, 11]. The platelets participate in many levels of the reaction sequence that produces fibrin thread and are component of the final clot structure, which comprise a fibrin mesh, with the activated platelet aggregate and red and white blood cell complex within. Since calcium ions are necessary for blood clotting, an effective agent capable of binding calcium ions or removing it from the environment prevents the progress of the coagulation process. Citrate, which binds to calcium ions and forms the calcium citrate molecule, is a soluble but unionizable substance. Classical blood preservatives include citrate dextrose and citrate phosphate dextrose as well as other substances to maintain cellular viability [9, 13–15].

3. Wound healing process

There are three overlapping stages to wound healing: inflammatory, proliferative, and remodeling. Inflammation is the first response to tissue damage. The goal is to provide rapid hemostasis and initiate a series of reactions leading to tissue regeneration. When blood exits from damaged vessels, a hematoma that fills the tissue space occurs, and platelets have crucial roles in this process. Cytokines and growth factors released from activated platelets and other cells result in several events, including cell migration, proliferation, differentiation, and matrix synthesis [16–19]. The fibrin mesh in the hematoma serves as a transient matrix to continue regenerative space and ensure a scaffold for migration and proliferation of cells [18, 20].

Neutrophils, inflammatory cells which first infiltrate the wound area and have lifetimes limited to hours and days, provide rapid defense against infections and removal of tissue debris. Then a flow of monocytes and T lymphocytes occurs to wound area [16, 17, 19, 21].

After monocytes reach the wound area, they differentiate into macrophages, and macrophages become predominant cell types in this region. The macrophages, which have lifetimes limited to days to months, support neutrophils in their functions and increase secretion of factors from neutrophils [16–18, 21]. The role of T lymphocytes in a successful wound healing process is still not clearly understood [19]. The mesenchymal stem cells migrate to the wound site to form an unstable cell line that will serve as a skeleton for or formation of the bone, cartilage, fibrous tissue, blood vessels, and other tissues [17]. Fibroblasts migrate to the wound site and begin to proliferate to produce extracellular matrix [17, 22]. Blood vessel endothelium close to the injury area proliferates to create new capillaries, and then these new vessels extend to the damaged site. These activities are regarded as the first steps of angiogenesis [16, 17].

During the proliferative phase, which is the second stage of wound healing, damaged and necrotic tissue is removed from the surrounding and replaced by living tissue that is in accordance with the original tissue structure of that region (e.g., bone, cartilage, fibrous tissue). Mesenchymal stem cells differentiate into fibroblasts, osteoblasts, chondrocytes, and other cell types which are required to produce the appropriate tissue type [17].

The third phase, the remodeling phase, is the final stage of wound healing. During this phase, the newly generated tissue reshapes and reorganizes to more closely resemble the original tissue [17].

4. Roles of platelets in wound healing

A lot of proteins are found within the alpha granules of platelets that strongly influence wound healing process, including transforming growth factor (TGF)-beta, platelet-derived growth factor (PDGF), platelet-derived endothelial growth factor (PDEGF), platelet-derived angiogenesis

Growth factor	Function in wound healing
Connective tissue growth factor (CTGF)	• Proliferation, migration, and tube formation of vascular endothelial cells and angiogenesis • Proliferation and differentiation of osteoblasts and matrix mineralization
aFGF or FGF-1 (fibroblast growth factor; acidic)	• Promotes skin-derived keratinocytes, dermal fibroblasts, and vascular endothelial cells • Participates in proliferation, differentiation, angiogenesis, and cell migration
bFGF or FGF-2 (fibroblast growth factor; basic)	• Promotes angiogenesis, endothelial cell proliferation, collagen synthesis, matrix synthesis, and epithelization • Growth of fibroblasts, myoblasts, osteoblasts, neural cells, endothelial cells, keratinocytes, and chondrocytes
GM-CDF or CSF a (granulocyte/ macrophage colony-stimulating factor)	• Chemoattractant for neutrophils • Participates in the proliferation and differentiation of osteoblasts and in the proliferation of BM progenitor cells
Insulin-like growth factor (IGF)	• Growth factors for normal fibroblasts, promotes the synthesis of collagenase and prostaglandin E2 in fibroblasts • Induces collagen and matrix synthesis by bone cells, regulating the metabolism of joint cartilage
Interleukin-1b (IL-1b)	• Activates osteoclasts in high concentrations and suppresses the formation of the new bone. In low concentrations, however, promotes new bone growth • Enhances inflammatory reactions and collagenase activity and inhibits the growth of endothelial cells and hepatocytes
Interleukin-8 (IL-8)	• Stimulates mitosis of epidermal cells and supports angiogenesis
Keratinocyte growth factor (KGF or FGF-7)	• Most potent GF for skin keratinocytes • Promotes wound healing via proliferation, differentiation, angiogenesis, and cell migration • Stimulates mitosis of epithelial cells except for fibroblasts and endothelial cells
Platelet-derived growth factor (PDGF)	• Activates TGF-b and stimulates neutrophils, macrophages, and mitosis of fibroblasts and smooth muscle cells, collagen synthesis, collagenase activity, and angiogenesis • Chemoattractant for hematopoietic and mesenchymal cells, fibroblasts, and muscle cells. Stimulates chemotaxis toward a gradient of PDGF
Transforming growth factor alpha (TGF-a)	• Affects bone formation and remodeling by inhibition of synthesis of collagen and release of calcium • More potent than EGF • Promotes the generation of osteoblasts and deposition of bone matrix during osteogenesis • Stimulates mesenchymal, epithelial, and endothelial cell growth. Endothelial chemotaxis controls the epidermal development
Transforming growth factor beta (TGF-b1)	• Fibroblast chemotaxis, proliferation, and stimulates collagen synthesis • Growth inhibitor for epithelial and endothelial cells, fibroblasts, neuronal cells, hematopoietic cell types, and keratinocyte
Tumor necrosis factor alpha (TNFa)	• Growth factor for fibroblasts and promotes angiogenesis
Vascular endothelial growth factor (VEGF/VEP)	• Induces neovascularization by stimulating the proliferation of macrovascular endothelial cells • Stimulates the synthesis of metalloproteinase that helps degrade interstitial collagen types 1, 2, and 3

Table 1. Growth factors in platelet and their function.

factor (PDAF), platelet factor 4 (PF4), vascular endothelial growth factor (VEGF), epidermal growth factor (EGF), epithelial cell growth factor (ECGF), insulin-like growth factor (IGF), interleukin (IL)-1, osteocalcin, osteonectin, vitronectin, fibrinogen, fibronectin, and thrombospondin (TSP)-1 [8, 11, 13, 16, 20, 21, 23, 24]. Collectively, these proteins mentioned are members of the growth factor, cytokine, and chemokine families. Each of these proteins takes a position in different steps of wound healing (**Table 1**) [9, 21]. Platelets begin to actively secrete these mediators within 10 minutes after clotting, and more than 95% of these presynthesized growth factors are secreted within 1 h [9, 21].

5. Platelet-rich plasma (PRP)

As a general definition, PRP is the concentration of autologous human platelets in a small amount of plasma. There are many different names, types, and PRP-like products (**Table 2**) [2–28]. PRP was first described by Marx et al. [2–28].

Some investigators have suggested that the platelet concentration in PRP should be at least 3–5 times the normal platelet concentration in the blood (**Table 3**) [29–32], although the dependence of clinical benefit on platelet concentration versus total number of platelets delivered may need to await further investigation [33]. Platelet concentration ratios of less than twofold to 8.5-fold have been reported [21, 29–31, 34–36]. Weibrich et al. [24] recommend that different individuals may need different platelet concentration ratios to obtain comparable biological effect.

PRP comprises not only high levels of platelets but also all components of clotting factors. For PRP to be clinically effective, it is emphasized that each 1 microliter of PRP should have at least 1,000,000 thrombocytes. (**Tables 3** and **4**) [29–32, 37].

Platelet-rich plasma (PRP)	Nonactivated plasma with amount of platelets above baseline
Platelet-rich fibrin (PRF)	Platelet-rich product with 3D structure
Platelet concentrate	Platelet-rich plasma
Plasma rich in growth factors	Type of pure PRP, no leukocytes
Platelet gel	Activated PRP
Platelet lysate	Activated PRP by lyses, e.g., by freeze-thawing or Triton-X
Platelet releasate	Activated PRP by thrombin and calcium chloride

Table 2. An overview of different names, types, and PRP-like products.

Thrombocytes baseline whole blood ($\times 10^9$/L)	519.6 ± 214.3
Thrombocytes PRP ($\times 10^9$/L)	2139.3 ± 1401.6
Ratio thrombocytes PRP/baseline whole blood	3.9 ± 1.8

Table 3. Platelets of the whole blood and PRP.

Growth factor	Physiologic level in the blood	Level in PRP
PDGF-β	3.3 ± 0.9 ng/ml	17 ± 8 ng/ml
TGF-β1	35 ± 8 ng/ml	120 ± 42 ng/ml
VEGF	155 ± 110 pg/ml	955 ± 1030 pg/ml
EGF	129 ± 61 pg/ml	470 ± 320 pg/ml

Table 4. Levels of some growth factors in blood versus PRP.

PRP acts through the degradation of alpha granules in the platelets. Secretion of growth factors begins from alpha granules within 10 min after clotting and more than 95% of the presynthesized growth factors secreted within 1 hour. In practice, after the PRP is prepared, it is necessary to induce the alpha granules in platelets for the release of growth factors. This induction is made by adding calcium and/or thrombin into PRP prepared in vitro. For this reason, the PRP should be prepared without clotting and should be applied within 10 minutes after clot initiation [9]. Basically, PRP is acquired by centrifuging autologous blood at a certain cycle. To keep the integrity of platelet membrane, acid citrate dextrose type A is used as anticoagulant agent [38].

While preparing the PRP, common points in clinical preparation techniques are like that: The blood is collected from the patient and is taken into the tube containing anticoagulant agent, and immediately centrifuge operation is initiated. When blood containing anticoagulant agent is centrifuged, three layers form as a result of the density: the deep layer containing red blood cells (gravity, 1.09), the middle layer containing white blood cells and platelets (buffy coat; gravity, 1.06), and the top layer (platelet poor plasma; gravity, 1.03) [11].

In the second stage, different techniques are applied, but basically, acellular plasma layer and the red cell layer are removed, and only "buffy coat" layer which contains dense platelet and white blood cells is obtained. So, the PRP becomes ready to be applied after addition of calcium and/or thrombin to activate thrombocytes [9].

Additionally, approximately 6 ml of platelet-rich plasma can be produced from 45 to 60 ml of blood thanks to newly developed small, compact office systems [14, 21, 39–41]. Numerous of such systems are available in use, including the PCCS (Implant Innovations, Inc., Palm Beach Gardens, Fla.), the Symphony II (DePuy, Warsaw, Ind.), the GPS (Biomet, Warsaw, Ind.), the Magellan (Medtronic, Minneapolis, Minn.), and the SmartPReP (Harvest Technologies Corp., Norwell, Mass.). Though, all these systems work on a small volume of obtained blood (45–60 ml) and on the principle of centrifugation, they have many differences in their capacity to collect and concentrate platelets, with about 30–85% of the available platelets collected and from a less than twofold to an approximately eightfold rise in the concentration of platelets over baseline [15, 30, 33, 35, 40, 42].

Although it is possible to produce PRP by using standard laboratory centrifuge, this process needs much effort, usually requiring multiple transfers and two spins; therefore, it may be difficult to maintain the sterility [14, 31, 43]. Moreover, these techniques may not be reliable to maximize platelet concentration or the levels of key secretory proteins [21].

PRP is stable, in the anticoagulated state, for up to 8 h after preparation. This duration allows to be used even during long operations [14, 21, 44]. In order to release the contents of alpha granules in the platelets, PRP must be activated. For this purpose, most commonly, 1000 units of topical bovine thrombin per milliliter of 10% calcium chloride solution is added to the platelet-rich plasma [16, 34, 39, 45].

6. PRP in wound healing

There are studies evaluating the effects of PRP on wound healing (**Table 5**) [37, 46, 47]. In the early phase of wound healing, the clot formed in the injury area serves as a matrix for cell migration, and this phase is primarily effected by platelets. Platelets contain over 1100 proteins, including growth factors, immune system mediators, enzymes, enzyme inhibitors, and bioactive compounds involved in the wound healing process. PRP contains important growth

Name	Type of wound	Method of use	Results
Almdahl et al.	Saphenous vein harvest site	PRP was sprayed on the wound before closure	No difference for the infection rate and cosmetic scale
Bahar et al.	Acute pilonidal abscess surgical site	The cavity was completely filled with PRP 24/36 h after surgery and covered with Vaseline gas	No healing time difference Significant difference for the test group on a pain relief scale and regarding the time to return to work
Kazakos et al.	Acute limb soft tissue wounds	Application of PRP gel once weekly	Significant difference for the test group regarding the time before reconstructive surgery by skin graft
Lawlor et al.	Surgical incisions for vascular surgery	PRP is sprayed during wound closure	No difference for the infection rate
Spyridakis et al.	Surgical excision of pilonidal sinus left opened for secondary healing	Application on the wound of PG on postoperative days 4 and 12	Significant difference for the test group regarding the complete healing time and quality of life
Han et al.	Full-thickness 5 mm punch wounds	Application on the wound	Significant difference for the test group regarding epithelialization at the tenth day
Hom et al.	Full-thickness 4 mm punch wounds	Application on the wound bed on postoperative days 0 and 7	Significant difference for test group regarding the healing time
Lee et al.	Full-thickness 2.5 × 2.5 cm skin wounds	Application on the wound	No difference regarding the healing rate
Molina-Minafio et al.	Full-thickness 6 mm punch wounds	Application on the wound	Significant difference for the test group regarding epithelialization at day 7 but not at day 28
Khalafi et al.	Sternal closure and saphenous vein harvest site	Application of PRP on the sternum, on the subcutaneous tissue, and on the wound edges	Significant difference for the test group regarding chest infection No difference regarding the saphenous vein harvest site infection rate Significant difference for the test group regarding chest and leg excessive drainage

Table 5. Some studies using PRP for wound healing.

factors deposited in alpha granules of platelets and plasma proteins such as fibrin, fibronectin, and vitronectin [37, 46, 47]. While plasma proteins serve as a skeleton for the bone, connective tissue, and epithelial migration, cocktail of growth factors plays an important role in tissue repair and regeneration. Degradation of previously stored growth factors occurs after contact with coagulation triggers such as collagen and tissue thromboplastin. Platelet activation with exogenous thrombin is associated with massive thrombin release and may reduce biological activity. Ten minutes after platelet activation, platelets start to deliver growth factors and give 95% of these molecules to environment in an hour [21]. Therefore, platelets should be applied within 10 min after activation. After release growth factors attach to mesenchymal stem cells, osteoblasts, fibroblasts, endothelial cells, and transmembrane receptors expressed by epidermal cells. The best known growth factors are platelet-derived growth factor, fibroblast growth factor, transforming growth factor beta, epidermal growth factor, vascular endothelial growth factor, and insulin-like growth factor. This attachment triggers the internal signaling pathway and leads to the expression of gene sequences that increase the normal wound healing process, such as cell proliferation, matrix formation, osteoid production, and collagen synthesis. Topical application of PRP accelerates the reepithelialization process by upregulating regulatory proteins of cell cycle such as cyclin A and CDK4. PRP is a potent matrix metalloproteinase (MMP)-1 stimulator and, thus, allows the extracellular matrix to be reorganized during wound healing [48, 49].

PRP may also suppress inflammation by suppressing cytokine release and increases regeneration and reepithelization by triggering capillary angiogenesis. The involvement of macrophages in the wound healing process is also mediated by signal proteins released from platelets. PRP has also been reported to exhibit antimicrobial activity against microorganisms such as *Escherichia coli*, MRSA, *Candida albicans*, and *Cryptococcus neoformans* and to have analgesic effect. Additionally, the pH 6.5–6.7 of the PRP may explain its antibacterial property. Although it has been suggested that leukocytes in PRP accelerate the recovery of soft tissue injury by suppressing bacterial growth, it has been also claimed that PRP may cause local pain and even suppress the healing process due to the inflammatory cytokines in it [50, 51].

In order for PRP therapy to be effective, it should contain 3–5 times the normal platelet level (approximately $0.8–1 \times 10^6/\mu L$). It is thought that, at very high platelet concentrations, it can suppress the wound healing with an opposite effect, because increase of the bioactive substances does not always mean a better effect. For example, at platelet concentrations higher than $1.5 \times 10^6/\mu L$, angiogenesis is suppressed. Eppley emphasizes that it is very difficult to achieve the desired platelet concentration because of the large number of variable and potential interactions [24, 35, 52].

A relation between growth factors in PRP with age and gender has not been detected. Since factors in PRP do not enter the cell or into the nucleus, it is assumed that there are no mitogenic or carcinogenic properties of PRP [46].

The use of PRP is contraindicated in coagulation defects (thrombocytopenia, anticoagulant use, hypofibrinogenemia), anemic situations, hemodynamic instability, and bovine thrombin hypersensitivity [53, 54].

7. PRP in burns

Growth factors play a crucial role in normal wound healing as well as impaired wound healing. Growth factors, such as insulin-like growth factor-1 (IGF-1) and platelet-derived endothelial cell growth factor (PDGF), inhibit apoptosis pathways which provide a rapid cell turnover and, thus, catalyze the physiologic wound healing in different steps. It is also thought that direct or indirect effects of growth hormone on wound healing are related to IGF-1 expression [55].

PRP is a new therapeutic option that is increasingly used especially in the treatment of soft and bony tissue defects to increase the tissue formation capacity and in improvement of chronic wound healing process [56–59]. Platelet-rich plasma, a rich source of growth factors released by activated platelets, is obtained from centrifuged blood which is combined with calcium chloride and thrombin [57, 58, 60].

Platelets are critical in the wound healing process and migrate to the wound site immediately and initiate coagulation when any damage occurs. Platelets are good sources of growth factors and cytokines associated with wound healing. Multiple growth factors and cytokines, including platelet-derived endothelial cell growth factor (PDGF), transforming growth factor-b (TGF-b1 and TGF-b2), transforming growth factor-a (TGF-a), platelet thromboplastin, thrombospondin, platelet-activating growth factor-4, vascular endothelial growth factor (VEGF), epidermal growth factor (EGF), coagulation factors, fibroblast growth factor (FGF), calcium, serotonin, histamine, and hydrolytic enzymes, with degranulation triggered by proteins such as thrombin are released by platelets [57, 58, 60].

Growth factors are key components of cellular activities related to wound repair. Growth factors mediate the migration of inflammatory cells into the wound site; they induce cell proliferation and differentiation and enhance extracellular matrix production and accumulation. Transforming growth factor beta is known to be an important mediator in tissue repair and has proven to be therapeutic in chronic nonhealing wounds [61, 62]. Platelet-derived endothelial cell growth factor promotes dermal regeneration, provokes protein and collagen synthesis that provides migration and angiogenesis, and increases TGF beta expression. Both transforming growth factor beta and platelet-derived endothelial cell growth factor are found at higher densities in PRP than platelet-poor plasma (PPP) [61].

Burn injury is a major reason of trauma that can result in death or disability, which requires a long recovery duration and high health care costs. In burn trauma, depth and size of burn injury, burn area, and patient age are the most important factors that affect the morbidity and mortality. Burn depth is also the most important parameter that determines the long-term appearance and functionality of the patient [63]. Conditions such as immunosuppression, extensive burn area, and malnutrition ensure an appropriate milieu for microorganisms, and unfortunately, infections are common and among the most important causes of morbidity and mortality in burn patients. Although the mortality rate is reduced with new treatment approaches in burn injuries, secondary infections and long recovery duration can still cause mortality. Early debridement and skin grafts can yield successful results, but inadequate graft donor area and unsuitable patient circumstances for surgery of burn patients are important obstacles for skin grafting [55, 62].

In these cases, using products that accelerate the wound healing process affects the morbidity and mortality of patients. Many different kinds of dressings or pharmacotherapies have been developed for this purpose, but these are very expensive, and mechanisms of action of these therapies are not fully documented [64–66]. Unfortunately, no optimal wound cover materials are currently available, but desired features of these materials include supporting increasing cells in wound healing, allowing vessel proliferation, keratinocyte adhesion, and differentiation and forming a barrier against fluid loss and microorganisms [62].

Platelet-rich plasma includes platelets, growth factors, cytokines, and clotting factors in high levels. Platelets in PRP initiate releasing these activated mediators in 10 min after clotting, and in the first hour, more than 95% of growth factors are released. Platelet-rich plasma stays stable, without losing its effectiveness, for approximately 8 h after preparation [57, 58]. PRP contain many different mediators, but TGF-b and PDGF are thought as the most important growth factors in PRP. They are involved in many stages of wound healing by triggering cell development and differentiation. Previous in vivo and in vitro studies have shown that cells which have roles in wound healing process are susceptible to growth factors [59]. Fibroblastatin is known to be sensitive to PDGFa, PDGFb, IGF, bFGF, and EGF [67]. Epidermal growth factor acts as a chemotactic factor for fibroblasts and, also, when administered topically enhances epidermal regeneration and strength of wound tension [59]. Endothelial cells are susceptible to VEGF and bFGF [68]. Growth factors such as VEGF, PDGF, and bFGF are triggers for vessel proliferation [69]. Fibroblast and smooth muscle cell migration and proliferation are induced by platelet-derived endothelial cell growth factor; also it is shown that PDGF is a chemotactic factor for neutrophils and monocytes and increases collagen deposition [60]. Additionally, PDGF and bFGF promote chondrocyte, osteoblast, and periosteal cell proliferation [70]. Transforming growth factor-b1 acts as a regulator for cell differentiation, proliferation, chemotaxis, and synthesis of some extracellular matrix proteins [60]. The effects of enhancing collagen synthesis, granulation tissue, and strength of wound tension of TGF-b1 were observed in animal studies [59, 71]. Another effect of TGF-b is the promotion of suprabasal cell proliferation and epidermal regeneration. Furthermore, TGF-b stimulates glycosaminoglycan, collagen, and fibronectin synthesis from fibroblasts. Transforming growth factor-b induces collagen synthesis and accelerates collagen maturation in the early period of wound healing. In addition, it is shown that using TGF-b with PDGF increases collagen deposition effects of TGF-b [60].

PRP has been shown to improve wound healing process in acute trauma wounds, incisional wounds, and chronic nonhealing wounds and is a beneficial agent in reconstructions of soft and hard tissues. Furthermore, PRP enhances differentiation of epithelial cell and collagen bundle organization. In PRP-treated wounds, the inflammatory phase of wound healing is shortened, and prolonged inflammation process is not seen. These effects of PRP reduce bacterial infections and scar formation [56, 57, 59, 60, 62, 71].

Effects of growth factors in PRP on wound healing and successful results obtained with PRP treatment in other types of wound lead to the use of PRP for burn treatment. Despite the paucity of the literature on PRP in burns (**Table 6**) [72], in theory, a dermal burn could benefit from PRP in several ways. First, hemostatic qualities of PRP could reduce perioperative blood

Name	Type of wound	Method of use	Results
Klosova et al.	Split-thickness skin graft on deep burns	Application of PG on the skin graft	PG accelerates reaching normal elasticity for split-thickness skin graft (no statistical analysis)
Maciel et al.	Burn with an iron	Application of PG on the wound and 3 days later	PG accelerates complete healing (no statistical analysis)
Henderson et al.	Ultrapulse CO_2 laser 232 cm burns	Application of PG	No difference regarding reepithelialization

Table 6. PRP in burns.

loss, as well as improve the take rate of the skin grafts by decreasing continued bleeding, functioning as a fibrin glue, as well as providing a well-vascularized bed for the meshed skin graft. Furthermore, the positive effects of PRP on wound healing, as seen in reports on PRP in in vitro models, chronic and acute wounds, could contribute to faster closure of mesh interstices, because PRP promotes vascular ingrowth and fibroblast proliferation and possibly reepithelialization. A deep dermal burn also could benefit from PRP through its hemostatic antimicrobial abilities [73–76].

The addition of PRP to the graft site has been shown to accelerate wound healing and enhance epithelialization and angiogenesis in split-thickness skin grafts and donor sites. Klosová et al. reported that combination of split-thickness skin grafting (STSG) and autologous platelet concentrate reversed the viscoelastic properties of scars to the plateau state more rapidly than areas treated with STSG alone [77–79].

In a recent study, it was demonstrated that PRP provided a quick repair of the extracellular matrix and its components in deep second-degree burn wounds in horses, and also, it was observed that two applications of PRP treatment accelerated formation of extracellular matrix during the first half of wound healing [80]. Additionally, Hao et al. reported that using PRP with acellular xenogeneic dermal matrix for treatment of deep second-degree burns decreased infection rate and increased wound healing [62, 81].

On the other hand, it is ambiguous whether results obtained in chronic and acute wounds could be applicable in burn injury wounds because a burn wound has a distinct physiological features than these wounds, including an enhanced inflammatory response, both systemic and local; increased edema; and a reduced perfusion secondary to hypercoagulability and microthrombus formation [82–84]. Patients affected by burn trauma are in a changed systemic physiological status [82, 84] when compared with the other healthy subjects in whom PRP mostly has been used and studied so far. It is generally recommended to withdraw blood before surgery to avoid activation of the platelets, but apparently this is not possible in burn patients, in whom platelets are already massively activated. It is known that platelets of burn patients show a distinct course in time, with a nadir at postburn day 3 followed by a reactive peak at postburn day 15, with a gradual return to normal values around postburn day. Several factors such as burn surface area, age, and sepsis influence this time course. There is little data about how burns or other traumas affect platelet and platelet function. In patients who have been exposed to trauma, it has been demonstrated that platelets were activated at least 72 h after injury and had an increased functionality in the first 48 h. This might affect the quality of PRP and the timing of its application in burn patients [76].

The long term effect of PRP on scar formation after burn injury is another important consideration and has not yet been evaluated comprehensively. There are plenty of growth factors released from the platelets and leukocytes in PRP, and some of these growth factors are chemotactic in recruiting inflammatory cells and a prolonged inflammation which could cause hypertrophic scar [85]. Furthermore, scar formation consists of series of complex events, and the effects of single growth factors in this process are still being unraveled. Among the growth factors, TGF-β1, TGF-β2, and platelet-derived growth factor are especially remarkable, because these factors are associated with hypertrophic and keloid scarring of normal skin wounds as well as in burn wounds. On the other hand, how PRP, a cocktail of many different growth factors, might influence scar formation remains to be seen. There are a limited number of publications on the development of hypertrophic scarring after the use of PRP in wound healing until now, and most of these publications are not related to burn trauma [76]. One of these studies is authored by Prochazka et al. They reported that while in burn patients treated with PRP combination, the rate of reepithelialization may not have been higher or faster than traditionally observed, the inflammatory markers normalized faster, providing the reepithelialized wound more stable. Because patients treated with PRP combination showed minimal cicatrization, they had high quality of healing without evidence of scar hypertrophy or contractures [76]. Additionally, recently some reports were published with positive results of PRP in combination with adipose cells for scar treatment; therefore, there might be an indication for PRP in the reconstructive aspect of burn treatment. On the other hand, in another study, long-term follow-up results did not show significant differences in scar quality in patients treated with PRP combination [86].

Furthermore, PRP treatment provides less pain and pruritus during the wound healing in burn trauma. And, one of the most important benefits of PRP in burn therapy is the cost-effectiveness of the therapy. The cost of hospital stay is lower (approximately 25% less) than that of patients who did not receive PRP combination treatment [87, 88].

Author details

Mehmet Unal

Address all correspondence to: dr.munal1101@gmail.com

Department of Dermatology and Venerology, Faculty of Medicine, Selcuk University, Konya, Turkey

References

[1] Fernandez-Moure JS, Van Eps JL, Cabrera FJ, Barbosa Z, Medrano Del Rosal G, Weiner BK, Ellsworth WA 4th, Tasciotti E. Platelet-rich plasma: A biomimetic approach to enhancement of surgical wound healing. The Journal of Surgical Research. 2017 Jan;**207**:33-44

[2] Marcus AJ. Platelet function. The New England Journal of Medicine. 1969;**280**:1278-1284

[3] Schapiro JM, Arber N, Sidi Y. Platelet hyperreactivity and prognosis in survivors of myocardial infarction. The New England Journal of Medicine. 1990;**323**:1707

[4] Dean WL, Lee MJ, Cummins TD, Schultz DJ, Powell DW. Proteomic and functional characterisation of platelet microparticle size classes. Thrombosis and Haemostasis. 2009;**102**:711

[5] White JG, Michelson A. Platelet structure. Platelets. 2007;**3**:117-144

[6] Oprea WE, Karp JM, Hosseini MM, Davies JE. Effect of platelet releasate on bone cell migration and recruitment in vitro. The Journal of Craniofacial Surgery. 2003;**14**:292-300

[7] Schober A, Manka D, von Hundelshausen P, et al. Deposition of platelet RANTES triggering monocyte recruitment requires P-selectin and is involved in neointima formation after arterial injury. Circulation. 2002;**106**:1523-1529

[8] Harrison P, Cramer EM. Platelet alpha-granules. Blood Reviews. 1993;**7**:52

[9] Epply BL, Pietrzak WS, Blanton M. Platelet-rich plasma. A review of biology and applications in plastic surgery. Plastic and Reconstructive Surgery. 2006;**118**:147e-159e

[10] Conley CL. Hemostasis. In: Mountcastle VB, editor. Medical Physiology. St. Louis: Mosby; 2004. p. 1137-1146

[11] Welsh WJ. Autologous platelet gel: Clinical function and usage in plastic surgery. Cosmetic Dermatology. 2000;**11**:13

[12] Caro CD, Pedley TJ, Schroter RC, et al. The Mechanics of the Circulation. Oxford: Oxford University Press; 1978

[13] Guyton AC. Physiology of the Human Body. Philadelphia: Saunders College Publishing; 1979

[14] Marx RE. Platelet-rich plasma (PRP): What is PRP and what is not PRP? Implant Dentistry. 2001;**10**:225

[15] Tischler M. Platelet rich plasma: The use of autologous growth factors to enhance bone and soft tissue grafts. The New York State Dental Journal. 2002;**68**:22

[16] Bhanot S, Alex JC. Current applications of platelet gels in facial plastic surgery. Facial Plastic Surgery. 2002;**18**:27

[17] Buckwalter JA, Einhorn TA, Bolander ME, et al. Healing of musculoskeletal tissues. In: Rockwood CA Jr, Bucholz RW, Green DP, editors. Fractures in Adults. Philadelphia: Lippincott-Raven; 1996. p. 261-304

[18] Anderson JM. The cellular cascades of wound healing. In: Davies JE, editor. Bone Engineering. Toronto: EM Squared Inc.; 2000. p. 81-93

[19] Szpaderska AM, Egozi EI, Gamelli RL, et al. The effect of thrombocytopenia on dermal wound healing. The Journal of Investigative Dermatology. 2003;**120**:1130

[20] Froum SJ, Wallace SS, Tarnow DP, et al. Effect of platelet-rich plasma on bone growth and osseointegration in human maxillary sinus grafts: Three bilateral case reports. The International Journal of Periodontics & Restorative Dentistry. 2002;**22**:45

[21] Marx RE. Platelet-rich plasma: Evidence to support its use. Journal of Oral and Maxillofacial Surgery. 2004;**62**:489

[22] Lowe HC, Rafty LA, Collins T, et al. Biology of platelet-derived growth factor. In: Canalis E, editor. Skeletal Growth Factors. Philadelphia: Lippincott Williams & Wilkins; 2000. p. 129-151

[23] Petrungaro PS. Using platelet-rich plasma to accelerate soft tissue maturation in esthetic periodontal surgery. The Compendium of Continuing Education in Dentistry. 2001;**22**:729

[24] Weibrich G, Kleis WK, Hafner G, et al. Growth factor levels in platelet-rich plasma and correlations with donor age, sex, and platelet count. Journal of Cranio-Maxillo-Facial Surgery. 2002;**30**:97

[25] Dohan Ehrenfest DM, Bielecki T, Del Corso M, Inchingolo F, Sammartino G. Shedding light in the controversial terminology for platelet-rich products: Platelet-rich plasma (PRP), platelet-rich fibrin (PRF), platelet-leukocyte gel (PLG), preparation rich in growth factors (PRGF), classification and commercialism. Journal of Biomedical Materials Research. Part A. 2010;**95**:1280-1282

[26] Dohan Ehrenfest DM, Rasmusson L, Albrektsson T. Classification of platelet concentrates: From pure platelet-rich plasma (P-PRP) to leucocyte- and platelet-rich fibrin (L-PRF). Trends in Biotechnology. 2009;**27**:158-167

[27] Everts PA, van Zundert A, Schönberger JP, Devilee RJ, Knape JT. What do we use: Platelet-rich plasma or plateletleukocyte gel? Journal of Biomedical Materials Research. Part A. 2008;**85**:1135-1136

[28] Anitua E, Sánchez M, Orive G. The importance of understanding what is platelet-rich growth factor (PRGF) and what is not. Journal of Shoulder and Elbow Surgery. 2011;**20**: e23-e24 author reply e24

[29] Marx RE. Platelet concentrate: A strategy for accelerating and improving bone regeneration. In: Davies JE, editor. Bone Engineering. Toronto: University of Toronto; 2000. p. 447-453

[30] Kevy SV, Jacobson MS. Comparison of methods for point of care preparation of autologous platelet gel. The Journal of Extra-Corporeal Technology. 2004;**36**:28

[31] Gonshor A. Technique for producing platelet-rich plasma and platelet concentrate: Background and process. The International Journal of Periodontics & Restorative Dentistry. 2002;**22**:547

[32] Marck RE, Gardien KL, Stekelenburg CM, Vehmeijer M, Baas D, Tuinebreijer WE, Breederveld RS, Middelkoop E. The application of platelet-rich plasma in the treatment of deep dermal burns: A randomized, double-blind, intra-patient controlled study. Wound Repair and Regeneration. 2016 Jul;**24**(4):712-720

[33] Waters JH, Roberts KC. Database review of possible factors influencing point-of-care platelet gel manufacture. The Journal of Extra-Corporeal Technology. 2004;**36**:250

[34] Marx RE, Carlson ER, Eichstaedt RM, et al. Platelet-rich plasma: Growth factor enhancement for bone grafts. Oral Surgery, Oral Medicine, Oral Pathology, Oral Radiology, and Endodontics. 1998;**85**:638

[35] Eppley BL, Woodell JE, Higgins J. Platelet quantification and growth factor analysis from platelet-rich plasma: Implications for wound healing. Plastic and Reconstructive Surgery. 2004;**114**:1502

[36] Weibrich G, Kleis WK, Kunz-Kostomanolakis M, et al. Correlation of platelet concentration in platelet-rich plasma to the extraction method, age, sex, and platelet count of the donor. The International Journal of Oral & Maxillofacial Implants. 2001;**16**:693

[37] Steed DL. The role of growth factors in wound healing. The Surgical Clinics of North America. 1997;**77**(3):575-586

[38] Zimmermann R, Jakubietz R, Jakubietz M, Strasser E, Schlegel A, Wiltfang J, et al. Different preparation methods to obtain platelet component as a source of growth factors for local application. Transfusion. 2001;**41**:1217-1224

[39] Man D, Plosker H, Winland-Brown JE. The use of autologous platelet-rich plasma (platelet gel) and autologous platelet-poor plasma (fibrin glue) in cosmetic surgery. Plastic and Reconstructive Surgery. 2001;**107**:229

[40] Marlovits S, Mousavi M, Gabler C, et al. A new simplified technique for producing platelet-rich plasma: A short technical note. European Spine Journal. 2004;**13**(Suppl. 1): S102

[41] Lozada JL, Caplanis N, Proussaefs P, et al. Platelet-rich plasma application in sinus graft surgery: Part I. Background and processing techniques. The Journal of Oral Implantology. 2001;**27**:38

[42] Arm DM. Autologous platelet-based therapies for orthopaedic tissue regeneration. Orthopedics. 2002;**25**:169

[43] Slater M, Patava J, Kingham K, et al. Involvement of platelets in stimulating osteogenic activity. Journal of Orthopaedic Research. 1995;**13**:655

[44] Anderson NA, Pamphilon DH, Tandy NJ, et al. Comparison of platelet-rich plasma collection using the Haemonetics PCS and Baxter Autopheresis C. Vox Sanguinis. 1991;**60**:155

[45] Robiony M, Polini F, Costa F, et al. Osteogenesis distraction and platelet-rich plasma for bone restoration of the severely atrophic mandible: Preliminary results. Journal of Oral and Maxillofacial Surgery. 2002;**60**:630

[46] Schmitz JP, Hollinger JO. The biology of platelet-rich plasma. Journal of Oral and Maxillofacial Surgery. 2001;**59**(9):1119-1121

[47] Bulbul Baskan E. Platelet rich plasma therapy in chronic wound healing. Turkiye Klinikleri Journal of Cosmetic Dermatology Special Topics. 2014;**7**(3):13-19

[48] Kim SA, Ryu HW, Lee KS, Cho JW. Application of platelet-rich plasma accelerates the wound healing process in acute and chronic ulcers through rapid migration and upregulation of cyclin A and CDK4 in HaCaT cells. Molecular Medicine Reports. 2013;**7**(2):476-480

[49] Shin MK, Lee JW, Kim YII, Kim YO, Seok H, Kim NI. The effects of platelet rich clot releasate on the expression of MMP-1 and type I collagen in human adult dermal fibroblasts: PRP is a stronger MMP-1 stimulator. Molecular Biology Reports. 2014;**41**(1):3-8

[50] Edelblute CM, Donate AL, Hargrave BY, Heller LC. Human platelet gel supernatant inactivates opportunistic wound pathogens on skin. Platelets. 2015;**26**(1):13-16

[51] Mei-Dan O, Mann G, Maffulli N. Platelet-rich plasma: Any substance to it? British Journal of Sports Medicine. 2010;**44**(9):618-619

[52] Sundman EA, Cole BJ, Fortier LA. Growth factor and catabolic cytokine concentrations are influenced by the cellular composition of platelet rich plasma. The American Journal of Sports Medicine. 2011;**39**(10):2135-2140

[53] Kumaran MS. Platelet rich plasma in dermatology: Boon or bane? Indian Journal of Dermatology, Venereology and Leprology. 2014;**80**(1):5-14

[54] Smith SE, Roukis T. Bone and wound healing augmentation with platelet rich plasma. Clinics in Podiatric Medicine and Surgery. 2009;**26**(4):559-588

[55] Poffenbarger PL, Haberal MA. Role of serum nonsuppressible insulin-like activity (NSILA) in wound healing. I. Influence of thyroparathyroidectomy on serum NSILA and wound healing in the rat. Surgery. 1976;**80**(5):608-616

[56] Iesari S, Lai Q, Rughetti A, Dell'Orso L, Clemente K, Famulari A, Pisani F, Favi E. Infected nonhealing wound in a kidney transplant recipient: Successful treatment with topical homologous platelet-rich gel. Experimental and Clinical Transplantation. 2017 Apr;**15**(2): 222-225

[57] Pallua N, Wolter T, Markowicz M. Platelet-rich plasma in burns. Burns. 2010;**36**(1):4-8

[58] Yol S, Tekin A, Yilmaz H, et al. Effects of platelet rich plasma on colonic anastomosis. The Journal of Surgical Research. 2008;**146**(2):190-194

[59] Kazakos K, Lyras DN, Verettas D, et al. The use of autologous PRP gel as an aid in the management of acute trauma wounds. Injury. 2009;**40**(8):801-805

[60] Carter CA, Jolly DG, Worden CE Sr, et al. Platelet-rich plasma gel promotes differentiation and regeneration during equine wound healing. Experimental and Molecular Pathology. 2003;**74**(3):244-255

[61] Knighton DR, Ciresi K, Fiegel VD, et al. Stimulation of repair in chronic, nonhealing, cutaneous ulcers using platelet-derived wound healing formula. Surgery, Gynecology & Obstetrics. 1990;**170**(1):56-60

[62] Ozcelik U, Ekici Y, Bircan HY, Aydogan C, Turkoglu S, Ozen O, Moray G, Haberal M. Effect of topical platelet-rich plasma on burn healing after partial-thickness burn injury. Medical Science Monitor. 2016 Jun 5;**22**:1903-1909

[63] Monstrey S, Hoeksema H, Verbelen J, et al. Assessment of burn depth and burn wound healing potential. Burns. 2008;**34**(6):761-769

[64] Fathke C, Wilson L, Hutter J, et al. Contribution of bone marrow-derived cells to skin: Collagen deposition and wound repair. Stem Cells. 2004;**22**(5):812-822

[65] Ichioka S, Kouraba S, Sekiya N, et al. Bone marrow-impregnated collagen matrix for wound healing: Experimental evaluation in a microcirculatory model of angiogenesis, and clinical experience. British Journal of Plastic Surgery. 2005;**58**(8):1124-1130

[66] Shakespeare PG. The role of skin substitutes in the treatment of burn injuries. Clinics in Dermatology. 2005;**23**(4):413-418

[67] Loot MA, Kenter SB, Au FL, et al. Fibroblasts derived from chronic diabetic ulcers differ in their response to stimulation with EGF, IGF-I, bFGF and PDGF-AB compared to controls. European Journal of Cell Biology. 2002;**81**(3):153-160

[68] Pintucci G, Froum S, Pinnell J, et al. Trophic effects of platelets on cultured endothelial cells are mediated by platelet-associated fibroblast growth factor-2 (FGF-2) and vascular endothelial growth factor (VEGF). Thrombosis and Haemostasis. 2002;**88**(5):834-842

[69] Go RS, Ritman EL, Owen WG. Angiogenesis in rat aortic rings stimulated by very low concentrations of serum and plasma. Angiogenesis. 2003;**6**(1):25-29

[70] Kaps C, Loch A, Haisch A, et al. Human platelet supernatant promotes proliferation but not differentiation of articular chondrocytes. Medical & Biological Engineering & Computing. 2002;**40**(4):485-490

[71] Ostvar O, Shadvar S, Yahaghi E, et al. Effect of platelet-rich plasma on the healing of cutaneous defects exposed to acute to chronic wounds: A clinico-histopathologic study in rabbits. Diagnostic Pathology. 2015;**10**:85

[72] Picard F, Hersant B, Bosc R, Meningaud JP. Should we use platelet-rich plasma as an adjunct therapy to treat "acute wounds," "burns," and "laser therapies": A review and a proposal of a quality criteria checklist for further studies. Wound Repair and Regeneration. 2015 Mar-Apr;**23**(2):163-170

[73] Kim DH, Je YJ, Kim CD, et al. Can platelet-rich plasma be used for skin rejuvenation? Evaluation of effects of platelet-rich plasma on human dermal fibroblast. Annals of Dermatology. 2011;**23**:424-431

[74] Graziani F, Ivanovski S, Cei S, Ducci F, Tonetti M, Gabriele M. The in vitro effect of different PRP concentrations on osteoblasts and fibroblasts. Clinical Oral Implants Research. 2006;**17**:212-219

[75] Carter MJ, Fylling CP, Parnell LK. Use of platelet rich plasma gel on wound healing: A systematic review and meta-analysis. Eplasty. 2011;**11**:e38

[76] Marck RE, Middelkoop E, Breederveld RS. Considerations on the use of platelet-rich plasma, specifically for burn treatment. Journal of Burn Care & Research. 2014 May-Jun;**35**(3):219-227

[77] Achora S, Muliira JK, Thanka AN. Strategies to promote healing of split thickness skin grafts: An integrative review. Journal of Wound, Ostomy, and Continence Nursing. 2014;**41**(4):335-339

[78] Kakudo N, Kushida S, Minakata T, et al. Platelet-rich plasma promotes epithelialization and angiogenesis in a split-thickness skin graft donor site. Medical Molecular Morphology. 2011;**44**(4):233-236

[79] Klosová H, Štětinský J, Bryjová I, et al. Objective evaluation of the effect of autologous platelet concentrate on post-operative scarring in deep burns. Burns. 2013;**39**(6):1263-1276

[80] Maciel FB, DeRossi R, Módolo TJ, et al. Scanning electron microscopy and microbiological evaluation of equine burn wound repair after platelet-rich plasma gel treatment. Burns. 2012;**38**(7):1058-1065

[81] Hao T, Zhu J, Hu W, et al. Autogenous platelet-rich plasma gel with acellular xenogeneic dermal matrix for treatment of deep II degree burns. Zhongguo Xiu Fu Chong Jian Wai Ke Za Zhi. 2010;**24**(6):647-649

[82] Shupp JW, Nasabzadeh TJ, Rosenthal DS, Jordan MH, Fidler P, Jeng JC. A review of the local pathophysiologic bases of burn wound progression. Journal of Burn Care & Research. 2010;**31**:849-873

[83] van de Goot F, Krijnen PA, Begieneman MP, et al. Acute inflammation is persistent locally in burn wounds: A pivotal role for complement and C-reactive protein. Journal of Burn Care & Research. 2009;**30**:274-280

[84] Evers LH, Bhavsar D, Mailänder P. The biology of burn injury. Experimental Dermatology. 2010;**19**:777-783

[85] van der Veer WM, Bloemen MC, Ulrich MM, et al. Potential cellular and molecular causes of hypertrophic scar formation. Burns. 2009;**35**:15-19

[86] Prochazka V, Klosova H, Stetinsky J, Gumulec J, Vitkova K, Salounova D, Dvorackova J, Bielnikova H, Klement P, Levakova V, Ocelka T, Pavliska L, Kovanic P, Klement GL. Addition of platelet concentrate to dermo-epidermal skin graft in deep burn trauma reduces scarring and need for revision surgeries. Biomedical Papers of the Medical Faculty of the University Palacky, Olomouc, Czech Republic. 2014 Jun;**158**(2):242-258

[87] Cervelli V, Nicoli F, Spallone D, et al. Treatment of traumatic scars using fat grafts mixed with platelet-rich plasma, and resurfacing of skin with the 1540 nm nonablative laser. Clinical and Experimental Dermatology. 2012;**37**:55-51

[88] Cervelli V, Palla L, Pascali M, De Angelis B, Curcio BC, Gentile P. Autologous platelet-rich plasma mixed with purified fat graft in aesthetic plastic surgery. Aesthetic Plastic Surgery. 2009;**33**:716-721

Chapter 7

Surgical Treatment of Burn Scars

Pertevniyal Bodamyalızade,
Emel Erdal Çalıkoğlu and Serap Maden

Additional information is available at the end of the chapter

http://dx.doi.org/10.5772/intechopen.72303

Abstract

The relationship between a burns patient and a reconstructive surgeon is normally long lasting and continues lifelong. Patients not only require a surgeon's professional expertise, but also time, optimism and compassion. Scar management relates to the physical and aesthetic components as well as the psychosocial implications of scarring. Hypertrophic scar formation which can cause debilitating deficiencies and poor aesthetic outcomes might be a result of burn injuries. Although nonsurgical treatment modalities in the early phase of scar maturation are critical to decrease hypertrophic scar formation, surgical management is often indicated to restore function. Operative scar management releases the tension and can often be achieved through local tissue arrangement.

Keywords: surgery, burn, scar, treatment

1. Introduction

Today, a lot of patients survive burn injuries, but they will not escape the burden of severe scar formation. The scarred tissue leaves contractures at joints, and this causes functional limitations. Surgical treatment is an indication to treat the burn scars [1]. In this chapter we explain the surgical treatment of burn scars.

Superficial burn wounds usually heal without complications. Deep partial and full-thickness burns have an increased risk for hypertrophic scar formation [2]. In the burns that include epidermis, the dermis remains intact and re-epithelization occurs by keratinocytes. Superficial partial-thickness burns involve epidermis and superficial dermis which results in blisters. Superficial injuries may require careful monitoring only. In deep partial-thickness burns, prolonged time for re-epithelialization is needed [3]. Assessing the depth of burn earlier is important to administer optimal treatment and prevent hypertrophic scar formation. Wound healing has three phases: inflammation, proliferation and remodeling [4, 5]. The dorsal area of the hands is thin and susceptible to hypertrophic scar formation. Dorsal scarring of the hands may not only inhibit passive flexion at the metacarpophalangeal joint but in some severe cases further result in hyperextension and subluxation of the joint [6].

A healed burn patient may have varying degrees of scars with functional and aesthetic components. Depending on the depth of the burn injury, post-burn scars are inevitable even with the best treatment. Second-degree deep dermal and full-thickness burns heal by scarring. The post-burn scars may be immature/mature, atrophic/hypertrophic/keloid, stable/unstable, depigmented (vitiligo)/hyperpigmented. They can turn into malignancy as well [7]. Unfortunately, the head and neck area are the most frequently affected area involved in burn injuries [8]. Especially, the neck with its ability to develop severe contractures and its aesthetic importance, deserves more attention [9]. Achieving long-term results with patient satisfaction remains a challenge [10]. Pre-expansion of free and regional axial island flap have all contributed to achieve this goal [11, 12]. The color match of skin grafts might be poor and also not as elastic as face and neck skin [13, 14]. Pre-expansion of tissue is valuable when large areas need to be resurfaced. This helps to cover more surfaces enabling the closure of the donor site. Studies showed that pre-expansion increases vascularization, reliability and the amount of tissue needed to be transferred [15–17]. Pre-expansion also causes atrophy of all expanded tissue layers except the epidermis that makes the flaps become thinner [18]. If there is no scar formation and the donor site can be closed primarily, then local options should be preferred. Supraclavicular flaps are preferred to infraclavicular flaps because they have greater proximity as well as better skin and tissue match to the affected areas when compared with infraclavicular flaps. Pre-expanded groin flaps show thinner dermis, expand easily and can be harvested without patient repositioning. If locoregional options cannot be used, in comparison to scapular and parascapular flaps, pre-expanded groin flaps are preferred (**Figure 1**).

As a rule, surgical treatment for post-burn contractures should not be undertaken during healing and scarring which usually takes 1 year. The surgical management of any post-burn contracture involves complete release of contracture. To decrease the requirement for skin cover, incision can be performed. To have a relatively bloodless field, incision line can be infiltrated with 1:200.000 adrenaline solution. The limb contractures can be released under tourniquet which should be deflated after complete release and hemostasis is achieved. Generally, for the patients who have received pre-operative physical therapy and their scars have become soft, incision rather than excision is applied to release the contracture. For example, in a case of post-burn contracture of neck, the scars may extend from chin, neck onto the chest and even abdomen. In this case, partial excision of hypertrophic scars may sometimes be done. If there is a contracture, it should be completely released. In severe long-standing contractures, the musculotendinous units and neurovascular structures can be shortened. Hence, complete release might be impossible. For example, if the joints are subluxated or dislocated, complete release might be impossible. In this case, the possible release is done, and then, full correction is achieved by serial splintage, skin/skeletal traction or by using the modern distractor systems. After the full correction is performed, then the skin is covered over the area. After releasing the contracture, the defect must be covered by using skin grafts or a skin flap [7].

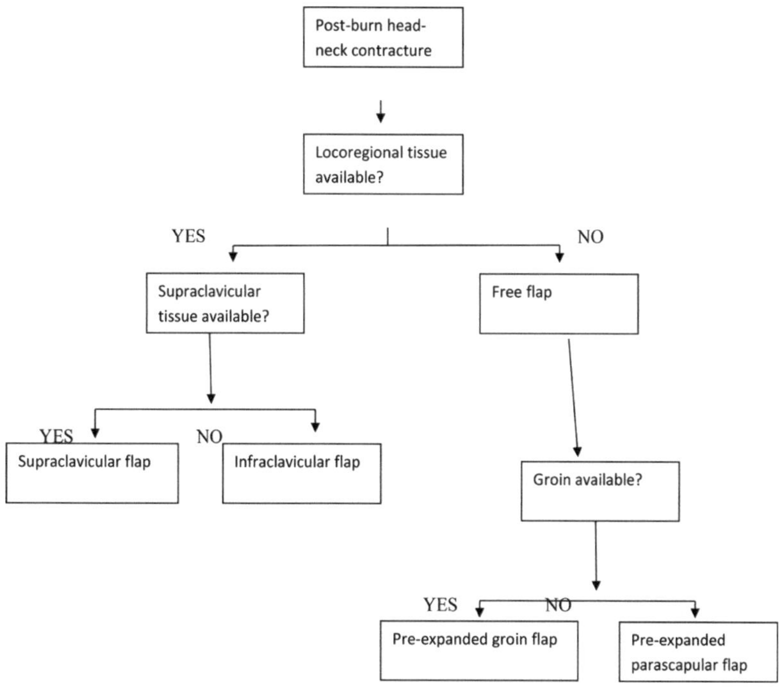

Figure 1. Post-burn treatment algorithm for head and neck contractures.

1.1. Skin graft

When we use the grafts sheet, grafts are preferred and expansion should not be preferred [13, 19, 20]. The junction line of the grafts' sheets should be parallel to the joint motion axis. After immediately release, the skin grafts are applied. Generally, contractures are treated with split skin grafts of intermediate or thick variety. This helps the donor site to heal up spontaneously.

1.2. Skin flaps

If the contracture release is likely to open up the joint of the hands and feet or tendon nerve, surgery is planned at a later date, for example, for old healed electrical burns, the skin flap is a must. The surgeon must provide a flap cover after release of contracture. If the defect is located in a cosmetic area and the reconstruction with a flap is thought to give a better cosmetic result, then covering a flap should be considered. For example, to repair upper lip ectropion of a male patient, the flap can be provided from scalp or upper neck. If it is a female patient, a graft cover is needed to repair upper lip ectropion.

1.3. Donor sites

For the split-skin grafts, thighs are usually used for harvesting. In a patient with severe burn and extensive scar formation, the grafts may be harvested from legs, abdomen and upper limb, scalp or back. In cases with multiple and massive contractures, the donor sites should be checked and plan charted out for "which donor site for which contracture." For neck, axilla and facial resurfacing, large sheets are important to be required while comparatively smaller pieces of graft are adequate for eyelid or finger contractures [7].

1.4. Postoperative care

The grafts become stable usually in 3 weeks time. Daily physical therapeutic exercises are required to keep the joints in range of motion. These exercises are continued till the grafts mature and range of motion is achieved. Care of the grafted areas is done till the graft loses its tendency to contract and can be pinched and moved over the recipient area [7]. According to Burn Association Repositories' data, it has been found that 500,000 burn victims seek medical treatment every year, and 39% of these injuries involve upper extremity and hand [2, 21, 22]. There are several risk factors for the formation of hypertrophic scars like young age, infection, skin stretch and anatomic location (axilla, neck) [23].

2. Operative burn scar management

In the acute phase of the thermal injury and during initial scar maturation, scar management can ameliorate hypertrophic scar formation and prevent scar banding. Timing of the operative procedure should allow enough time for complete scar maturation, as premature intervention can result in increased inflammation and additional scarring. Reconstructive procedures usually start 6 months after injury. For the correction of mild and moderate hypertrophic scar contractures, local skin flaps are commonly used to avoid more complex procedures [24]. Simple linear scar bands which can be seen across joints can be treated best with a scar-lengthening Z-plasty. The classic Z-plasty is designed with its central limb along the hypertrophic scar band and with a 60° angle of the lateral limbs. By making the corner 90° before extending the Z-plasty to 60°, perfusion to the tip of the Z-plasty is improved [25]. The flaps can be raised in scar tissue if maintained thick and involving underlying adipose tissue to achieve active lengthening of 75%. Creating the angle to 90° results in lengthening of 125%, however, involves larger limbs. To modify this approach, a series of smaller z-plasties along a scar can be performed. This helps to achieve similar lengthening but avoiding donor site morbidity with larger flaps. While larger flaps are used for axillary contractures, smaller flaps are used for palms and digits [26]. In web space contractures, modifications of plasties and a variety of local flaps are commonly devised [27, 28]. Because of its geometric design, the 5-flap Z-plasty is frequently used to create concavity and lengthening within the web space. Another option is the V-Y advancement flaps that use the supple dorsal tissue which is advanced into web space. These flaps can later on be combined with forms of z-plasties [29]. The second most common contractures behind neck contractures are the axillary scar contractures and they are difficult to improve. With z-plasties, small linear bands can be removed. Larger contractures can be treated with release and thick split thickness skin graft or full-thickness skin graft. Ogawa et al. describe treatment of severe contractures with pedicled flaps or with regional and free tissue transfer [30]. Usually palmar burn scars involve a large surface and result in tight contractures. Mild forms can be treated with a sequence of z-plasties. If it is a severe contracture, release of the scar may be required leaving a large defect. Full-thickness skin graft can be used to fill this defect. Full-thickness skin grafts are preferred over split-thickness graft because they have a decreased effect of secondary contraction to minimize scarring. If the contracture release leads to exposed tendon or bone, local flaps may be used [31].

2.1. General principles of contracture release

1. Proximal joint contractures should be released before distal contractures. For example, if the shoulder and elbow have limited range of movement, then there is a little value to have a mobile wrist.
2. If there are multiple joints requiring release, each joint should be considered separately and each contracture should be fully released. The Y-V plasty technique simultaneously leads to release of multiple joints.
3. Function is always prior over cosmesis; it is better to have a functioning joint with an albeit disappointing cosmesis than to have a cosmetically perfect joint without mobility. This does not mean cosmesis is not important but it should not take precedence over function.
4. When split-thickness graft is applied over a wound, it will again contract with the potential for recurrent contracture formation. To prevent this, physiotherapy is a method to mobilize the joint. A flap is much more preferred than a split-skin graft. It has its own blood supply and also supplies bulk, which might lead to better cosmetic appearance.
5. Sometimes, the important underlying structures may be exposed and require release. For example, a dorsal release of the ankle joint may leave extensor tendons exposed. In a long-standing contracture, ligaments and tendons may have permanently shortened, and tendon lengthening may be necessary for dorsiflexion.

2.2. Time for surgical contracture release

Burn contracture release is undertaken once it is deemed "mature." Interfering with an active scar leads further contracture formation. Contracture and hypertrophic scar formation increases in the first 6 months, and full scar maturation will occur after 2 years. When the scar is active, it is pliable and amenable to stretching by physiotherapy [32].

To reconstruct the contracture, surgical treatment should be combined with release and split-skin grafting. This recently is called conventional waiting approach. For example, in the acute lower lid treatment, some studies showed that full-thickness grafts reduce the incidence of subsequent ectropion release [33]. It is important that, when flap cover of the defect is planned, this timing restriction is not applicable. Some authors support waiting for 2 or 3 weeks acutely, prior to undertaking release and free flap cover, and have reported success rates of 94% [34].

2.3. How to treat the burn scar contractures

1. Split-skin grafting
2. Local plastic surgical procedures

a. Z-plasty

b. Y-V plasty

3. Full-thickness skin grafting

4. Flap cover

5. Artificial skin substitutes

6. Tissue expansion with or without flap cover

When there is a mild contracture which means that there is 50% of joint movement possibility, to lengthen the scar, Z-plasty can be performed. In more severe cases, different surgical procedures are needed.

To remove the contracture, even a band or a sheet of scar tissue must be fully released. Unless local adjacent skin flaps are used, the release and the reconstruction can be considered as two different procedures, e.g., Z-plasty. The contracture release incision must be placed at the meridian of the joint and must be "fish-mouthed" at either end, and should extend into normal tissue medially and laterally. Using a swab on the index finger will "sweep" tissue away from the center contracture and divide "softer" bands. By using this manoeuvre, the extent of the defect to be covered will be increased. It is also designed to be sure that the wound is formed from normal tissue, not scar.

2.3.1. Split-skin grafting

This traditional method of split-skin grafting helps the defect import non-scarred, healthy, non-bulky skin without the need to compromise local tissues. The graft is ideally harvested from buttocks or scalp, which are cosmetically acceptable sites [35]. Once the contracture is fully released and full joint extension is achieved, then the graft is only applied to the wound bed. The ability to release multiple joints at the same sitting is an advantage, but leading to hypertrophic scar formation is a disadvantage. Also, when a split-skin graft is placed on a wound bed, the wound will again contract and recurrence might occur and re-release can be required again.

Because there is a risk such as immobilization difficulty, bleeding and infection, the split-skin grafts are at risk of suboptimal "take." Then the patient needs physiotherapy for motion of joint especially in children. Donor site morbidity is also a problem.

2.3.2. Local surgical procedures

2.3.2.1. Z-plasty

If there is a contracture which is due to a band, then a "local" procedure which both divides the contracting band and lengthens it is amenable avoiding the need for a donor site. The Z-plasty is a technique that divides the scar contracture and lengthens the band by importing local lateral adjacent tissue. Z-plasty does not create new tissue to lengthen

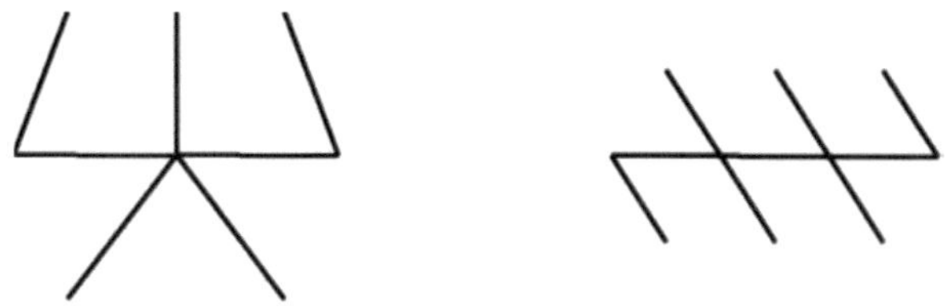

Figure 2. Z-plasty in series (5-flap Z-plasty); Z-plasty in parallel (multiple Z-plasties).

the band, but borrows tissue adjacent to the contracture. Unless there is a short contracture band with a good deal of lax adjacent skin, Z-plasty is possible. These can be thought of as Z-plasty-in-parallel or Z-plasty-in-series [36]. The Z-plasty-in-series (e.g., five-flap Z-plasty) recruits a large amount of adjacent tissue. The Z should always be designed as large as possible. The bigger the Z-plasty is in size, the greater the lengthening obtained. When compared the Z-plasty-in-parallel (e.g., multiple single Z-plasties) recruits much less adjacent tissue than Z-plasty-in-series. The actual lengthening obtained is relatively less (**Figure 2**).

If the surrounding tissue is less pliable, this technique can be used. There is a risk of ischemic necrosis when the undermining and subsequent transposition of skin flaps are in an area of scarring and fibrosis (especially the tips). The reorientation of the scar can also result in distortion of the surrounding tissues.

2.3.2.2. Y-V plasty

Y-V plasty is especially useful in linear sheet contractures. The V extends the whole length of the band, and the Y passes into normal skin. The scar is not excised. The flaps simply are pulled forward to form a V [37]. To achieve this, skin laxity should be enough [38], and the "pinch" test is useful to evaluate this [39].

The advantages of this technique:

1. There is little risk of flap tip necrosis because the blood supply of the flaps is less compromised as there is no need for undermining.

2. This technique effects reorientation of scar tissue.

3. The contracture band length is not important. This technique is especially useful in very long contracture bands. The running Y-V plasty is especially useful in these cases.

4. 100% lengthening of the long axis of the contracture which is the theoretical lengthening of the contracture [38].

This is only true when the flap can be advanced half the length of the sides of the V forming the flap. For two reasons, the actual lengthening obtained is much less than it is supposed to be. The first reason is as the burnt tissue has lost its elasticity, it is often difficult to advance the burnt skin. The second reason is interdigitation of each adjacent advancement flap. While using the "straight-line" advancement flaps, the problem is that the stretching of the skin limits the actual obtained lengthening. That is the reason only Y-V technique can be applied in mild contractures.

5. Y-V plasty is a simple procedure. While the operation is performed, the flap advancement degree can be refined. There is a disadvantage of this technique. Excision of a thick scar band is not actually possible, and there are poor cosmetic results (**Figure 3**).

The W-plasty, double-reverse V-Y plasty [40] and X-plasty [41] are the variations of the methods described above. To remove web-shaped burns, the seven-flap plasty has been described [42].

2.3.3. Full-thickness skin grafting

After the contracture release is complete, reconstruction with full-thickness grafting has a better texture match than with split-skin grafting, and is associated with less recurrence [13]. A full-thickness graft provides less wound contraction, because it has more dermis in the graft. After large burns, there may be limited available skin; thus in such cases, full-thickness grafts are impractical. Taking graft is much more tenuous than with split-skin grafts, when a contour to the underlying bed is required, like whole cheek, which is not a flat surface. Full-thickness grafts need a healthy bed on which to take and leave a donor site. They usually exhibit hyperpigmentation which causes poor cosmetic results.

2.3.4. Flap cover

Flap cover can be either a pedicled flap or free flap. To release the burn contracture, both local [43] and free [44] fasciocutaneous flaps are successfully used. In most of the superficial burns, perforators to the deep fascia are usually protected. In this case, a burn scar may itself be used as part of this flap [43]. In large burn areas, local pedicled flaps are sometimes inappropriate, however, due to the lack of local skin plasticity or simply a paucity of available or acceptable donor sites. In this situation, using a free flap should be considered. The latissimus dorsi, serratus anterior, lateral arm, scapular, gracilis, anterolateral thigh, arterialised venous

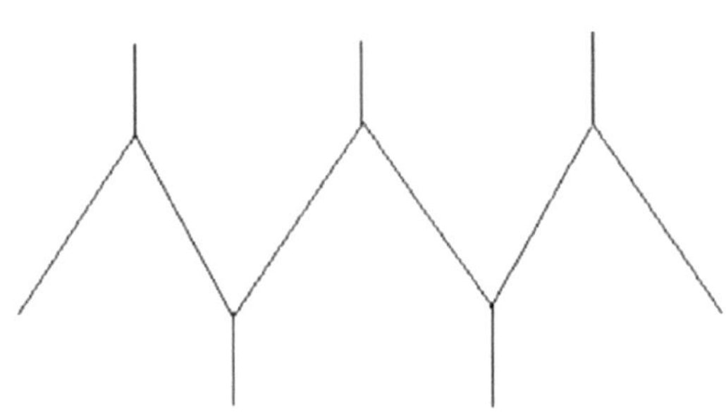

Figure 3. Y-V plasty. V is marked along the contracture band and Y extension passes into normal tissue on each side.

and temporalis fascial flaps are generally used [34]. There is a wide variety of flap choice which allows the surgeon to make judgments according to each individual case. There is no risk for recurrence, and this is the key advantage of flap. Free flaps may lead to an unacceptable cosmetic result because they import tissue different in color, thickness and texture. The flaps size must be as the same size as the defects size. Free flaps lead to a large donor defect and often require themselves a covering split-skin graft. Usually the adjacent tissue is burnt and the thick hypertrophic nature of the scar may make dissection of the recipient vessel difficult. Microvascular circulation should be kept up at higher level. Post-operative complications including complete or partial failure are disastrous. The free flap is an expensive and demanding procedure. It is a good option to apply when only one joint has a severe contracture from broad sheet of scar in the extremities.

2.3.5. Artificial skin substitutes

Following Yannas and Burke's original design, artificial skin templates have been developed [45]. Integra is a bilayer artificial dermis product consisting of porous bovine collagen spongy matrix combined with an overlying temporary epidermal substitute comprised of a silicone sheet. Combination of bilayer artificial dermis with split-skin grafting has been used by Soejima to reconstruct burn contractures [35]. The skin quality resembles full-thickness skin and also there is improved flexibility and suppleness, and scar hypertrophy does not exist [46]. There is reduced inflammatory response accompanying artificial skin substitutes, thus leading to reduced contraction. Donor site morbidity from split skin graft harvesting lower take rates than conventional autografts, more intensive dressing requirements and higher cost implications are the disadvantages [47]. This procedure has two steps. Sometimes it is noticed that areas of keloid scarring (and joint extremities in children) do not give good response to artificial dermis and tend to lead to recontracture or hypertrophic scar formation [35]. Hunt et al. treated a small series of neck contractures with Integra and they all developed recontracture [48]. The results of Integra over joints are disappointing despite adequate splintage [46]. In the management of complex wounds, Integra has been successful, but contamination and subsequent infection can lead to adverse results. A multicenter post-approval study in the United States including 216 burn injury patients found that the total incidence of infection in Integra-treated sites was 16.3% [49]. Another multicenter study managed with Integra following release of scar contractures noted a 20% infection rate. The second most common complication underneath Integra was fluid collection with 14% [50]. Matriderm is a thin (1 mm) single layer dermal matrix composed of collagen types I, III, and V and it has been marketed as a single-stage dermal template for reconstruction [51].

2.3.6. Expansion of tissue with or without flap cover

Expansion of tissue is a simple procedure. The color, texture and thickness of the expanded skin is the same as adjacent skin. Tissue expanders together with a pre-expanded free [52] or fasciocutaneous flap [53] can be used in contractures caused by burns. Expansion of tissues helps the maximum utilization of the non-involved areas.

The number of new scars and donor site morbidity is reduced. Neck, chest and scalp are the most suitable areas where tissue expansion is commonly performed. In the lower limb, expansion is especially difficult in the burned extremity [54]. While planning the expansion, it is often difficult to predict the size of the defect. Expansion has the risks of infection, leakage and skin ischemia, and even failure. The patients should attend regular follow-up to improve outcomes and reduce complication rates.

3. Clinical assessment

1. Is the reason for the contracture an intrinsic force or an extrinsic force?

   For example, if there is a burn scar on the cheek, then lower lid ectropion can occur without any intrinsic lower eyelid deformity.

2. How is the severity of the contracture? Is the joints range of motion more than 50%?
3. Is the cause of the contracture a broad sheet of scar or a band of scar?
4. What is the cause of the contracture? If it is a band, then is it surrounded by normal tissue or a burned tissue?
5. Check if the band includes only one joint or if it involves other joints.

Below, there is an algorithm to help surgeons to choose the best reconstruction process for burn contractures after release (**Figures 4** and **5**) [32].

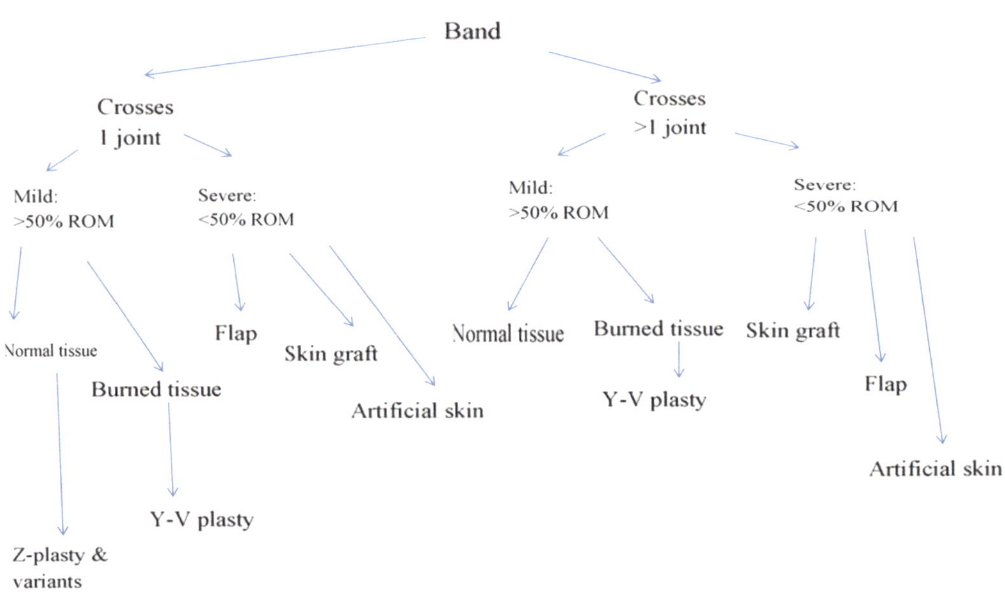

Figure 4. Algorithm for the cover of burn contractures of the extremities after release: band contracture (ROM = range of motion).

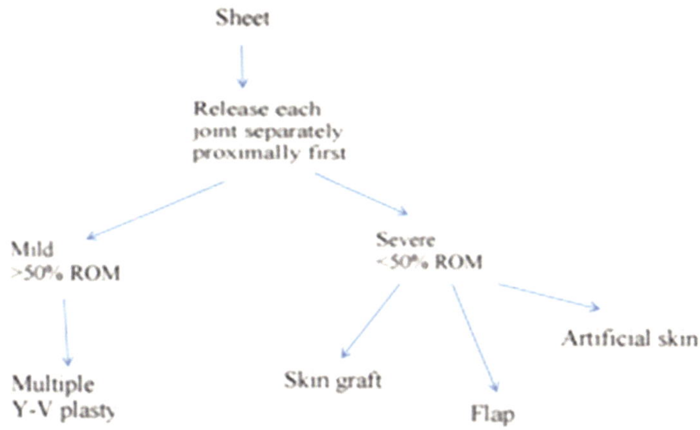

Figure 5. Algorithm for the cover of burn contractures of the extremities after release: broad sheet of scar (ROM = range of motion).

4. Conclusion

The algorithms above are an attempt to simplify the approach to burn contracture release. Naturally, there are situations where the algorithm might not be applicable, and the surgeon, in all such cases, must plan an approach according to knowledge and experience.

Author details

Pertevniyal Bodamyalızade, Emel Erdal Çalıkoğlu and Serap Maden

Address all correspondence to: pniyal@gmail.com

Near East University Hospital, Faculty of Medicine, North Nicosia, Northern Cyprus

References

[1] Stekelenburg CM, Mark RE, Verhaegen PDHM, et al. Perforator-based flaps for the treatment of burn scar contractures: A review. Burns & Trauma. 2017;**5**:5

[2] McKee DM. Acute management of burn injuries to the hand and upper extremity. Journal of Hand Surgery. 2010;**35**(9):1542-1544

[3] Monstrey S, Hoeksema H, Verbelen J, et al. Assesment of burn depth and burn wound healing potential. Burns. 2008;**34**(6):761-769

[4] Kwan P, Hori K, Ding J, et al. Scar and contracture: biological principles. Hand Clinics. 2009;**25**(4):511-528

[5] Tredget EE, Levi B, Donelan MB. Biology and principles of scar management and burn reconstruction. The Surgical Clinics of North America. 2014;**94**(4):793-815

[6] Graham TJ, Stern PJ, True MS. Classification and treatment of postburn metacarpophalangeal jointextension contractures in children. Journal of Hand Surgery. 1990;**15**(3):450-456

[7] Goel A, Shrivastava P. Post-burn scars and scar contractures. Indian Journal of Plastic Surgery. 2010;**43**(Supplement 1)

[8] Prasad JK, Bowdwn ML, Thomson PD. A review of the reconstructive surgery need of 3167 survivors of burn injury. Burns. 1991;**17**:302-305

[9] Edlich RF, Nichter LS, Persing JA. Burns of the head and neck. Otolaryngologic Clinics of North America. 1988;**12**:361-388

[10] Angrigiani C. Aesthetic microsurgical reconstruction of anterior neck burn deformities. Plastic and Reconstructive Surgery. 1994;**93**:507-518

[11] Ninkovic M, Moser-Rumer A, Ninkovic M, et al. Anterior neck reconstruction with pre-expanded free groin and scapular flaps. Plastic and Reconstructive Surgery. 2004;**113**: 61-68

[12] Pallua N, von Heimburg D. Pre-expanded ultra-thin supraclavicular flaps for (full-) face reconstruction with reduced donor-site morbidity and without the need for microsurgery. Plastic and Reconstructive Surgery. 2005;**115**:1837-1844

[13] Iwuaqwu FC, Wilson D, Bailie F. The use of skin grafts in postburn contracture release: A 10-year review. Plastic and Reconstructive Surgery. 1999;**103**:1198-1201

[14] Voinchet V, Bardot J, Echinard C. Advantage of early burn excision and grafting in treatment of burn injuries of the anterior cervical region. Burns. 1995;**21**:126-128

[15] Argenta LC. Controlled tissue expansion in reconstructive surgery. Plastic and Reconstructive Surgery. 1990;**86**:520-529

[16] De Filippo RE, Atala A. Stretch and growth: The molecular and physiologic influences of tissue expansion. Plastic and Reconstructive Surgery. 2002;**109**:2450-2462

[17] Cherry GW, Austad E, Pasyk K, et al. Increased survival and vascularity of random pattern skin flaps elevated in controlled, expanded skin. Plastic and Reconstructive Surgery. 1983;**72**:680-687

[18] Van Rappard JH, Sonneveld GJ, Borghouts JM. Histologic changes in soft tissues due to tissue expansion (in animals studies and humans). Facial Plastic Surgery. 1998;**5**:280-286

[19] Harrison CA, MacNeil S. The mechanism of skin graft contraction: An update on current research and potential future therapies. Burns. 2008;**34**:153-163

[20] Rudulph R, Ballantyne DL. Skin Grafts. In: McCarthy JG, editor. Plastic Surgery. Vol. 1. Philadelphia: W.B. Saunders Co; 1990. pp. 221-274

[21] Ng D, Anastakis D, Douglas LG, et al. Work-related burns: A 6 year retrospective study. Burns. 1991;**17**(2):151-154

[22] Sheridan RL, Hurley J, Smith MA, et al. The acutely burned hand: Management and outcome based on a ten year experience with 1047 acute hand burns. The Journal of Trauma. 1995;**38**(3):406-411

[23] Butzelaar L, Ulrich MM, Mink van der Molen AB, et al. Currently known risk factors for hypertrophic skin scarring: A review. Journal of Plastic, Reconstructive & Aesthetic Surgery. 2016;**69**(2):163-169

[24] Hop MJ, Langenberg LC, Hiddingh J, et al. Reconstructive surgery after burns: A 10-year follow-up study. Burns. 2014;**40**(8):1544-1551

[25] Rohrich RJ, Zbar RI. A simplified algorithm for the use of Z-plasty. Plastic and Reconstructive Surgery. 1999;**103**(5):1513-1517 [quiz: 1518]

[26] Sorkin M, Cholok D, Levi B. Scar management of the burned hand. Hand Clinics. 2017

[27] Sari E, Tellioglu AT, Altuntas N, et al. Combination of rhomboid flap and double Z-plasty technique for reconstruction of palmar and dorsal web space burn contractures. Burns. 2015;**41**(2):408 12

[28] Grishkevich VM. First web space post-burn contracture types: Contracture elimination methods. Burns. 2011;**37**(2):338-347

[29] Peker F, Celebiler O. Y-V advancement with Z-plasty: An effective combined model for the release of postburn flexion contractures of the fingers. Burns. 2003;**29**(5):479-482

[30] Ogawa R, Hyakusoku H, Murakami M, et al. Reconstruction of axillary scar contractures–retrospective study of 124 cases over 25 years. British Journal of Plastic Surgery. 2003;**56**(2):100-105

[31] Karanas YL, Buntic RF. Microsurgical reconstruction of the burned hand. Hand Clinics. 2009;**25**(4):551-556

[32] Hudson DA, Renshaw A. An algorithm for the release of burn contractures of the extremities. Burns. 2006;**32**:663-668

[33] Lille ST, Engrav LH, Caps MT, Orcutt JC, Mann R. Full-thicknessgrafting of acute eyelid burns should not be considered taboo. Plastic and Reconstructive Surgery. 1999;**104**(3):637-645

[34] De Lorenzi F, van der Hulst R, Boeckx W. Free flaps in burn reconstruction. Burns. 2001;**27**:603-612

[35] Soejima K, Nozaki M, Sasaki K, Takeuchi M, Negishi N. Reconstruction of burn deformity using artificial dermis combined with thin splitskin grafting. Burns. 1997;**23**:501-504

[36] Hudson DA. Some thoughts on choosing a Z-plasty: The Z made simple. Plastic and Reconstructive Surgery. 2000;**106**(3):665-671

[37] Ebbehoj J. Y to V instead of Z to N. Burns. 1983;**10**:121

[38] Lai CS, Lin SD, Tsai CC, Tsai CW. Running Y–V plasty for burn scar contracture. Burns. 1995;**21**:458-462

[39] Cooper MACS. The multiple Y–V plasty in linear burn scar contracture release. British Journal of Plastic Surgery. 1990;**43**:145-149

[40] Askar I. Double-reverse V–Y plasty in postburn scar contractures: A new modification of V–Y plasty. Burns. 2003;**29**(7):721-725

[41] Vartak A, Keswani MH. X-plasty for repair of burn contractures. Burns. 1992;**18**(4):326-328

[42] Suliman MT. Experience with the 7 flap-plasty for the release of burns contractures. Burns. 2004;**30**(4):374-379

[43] Hallock GG. The role of local fasciocutaneous flaps in total burn wound management. Plastic and Reconstructive Surgery. 1992;**90**(4):629-635

[44] Mast BA, Douglas Newton E. Aggressive use of free flaps in children for burn scar contractures and other soft tissue deficits. Annals of Plastic Surgery. 1996;**36**:569-575

[45] Yannas IV, Burke JF. Design of artificial skin. I. Basic design principles. Journal of Biomedical Materials Research. 1980;**14**:65-81

[46] Young RC, Burd A. Paediatric upper limb contracture release following burn injury. Burns. 2004;**30**:723-728

[47] Heimbach D, Luterman A, Burke J, et al. Artificial dermis for majorburns: A multi-center randomized clinical trial. Annals of Surgery. 1988;**208**:313-320

[48] Hunt JA, Moisidis E, Haertsch P. Initial experience of Integra in thetreatment of post-burn anterior cervical neck contracture. British Journal of Plastic Surgery. 2000;**53**(8):652-658

[49] Heimback DM, Warden GD, Luterman A, et al. Multicenter postapproval clinical trial of Integra dermal regeneration template for burn treatment. The Journal of Burn Care & Rehabilitation. 2003;**24**:42-48

[50] Frame JD, Still J, Lakhel-LeCoadou A, et al. Use of dermal regeneration template in contracture release procedures: A multicenter evaluation. Plastic and Reconstructive Surgery. 2004;**113**:1330-1338

[51] Theodore TN, Chiang HA, Leavitt T, Ozambela M, Orgill DP. Plastic and reconstructive surgery. Tissue-Engineered Skin Substitutes. Regenerative Medicine. December 2015;**136**(6):1379-2015

[52] Santanelli F, Grippando FR, Ziccardi P, Onesti MG. The role of preexpanded free flaps in revision of burn scarring. Burns. 1997;**23**(7-8):620-625

[53] Stuffer M, Papp C. Reconstruction of large scar areas with controlled skin expansion combined with fasciocutaneous flaps. Burns. 1991;**17**(2):166-169

[54] Pisarski GP, Mertens D, Warden GD, Neale HW. Tissue expansion complications in the paediatric burns patient. Plastic and Reconstructive Surgery. 1998;**102**:1008-1012